Intermittent Fasting For Women

A Complete Guide for Weight Loss, Managing Intermittent Fasting to Detox Body and Support Hormones

Thomas Felling

1

TABLE OF CONTENTS

Introduction

Intermittent fasting is a hot topic in eating and weight loss lately (everybody from Hoda Kotb has done it to Jennifer Aniston), but the principle itself is not unique. In fact, going without eating or drinking temporarily comes from the traditions of many major religions and cultures around the world. It consists of alternating fasting and eating cycles. Several studies have shown that this can lead to weight loss, improve metabolic health, protect against disease, and maybe allow you to live longer.

The book is all about intermittent fasting for women. Let me tell you first what intermittent fasting means actually. Intermittent fasting is a pattern of eating where you cycle between eating and fasting periods. It generally describes a simple concept: you can eat almost anything you want, but only for a certain period of time. It doesn't say anything about what foods to eat, but when to eat it. There are several intermittent methods of fasting, all dividing the day or week into periods of eating and fasting. Every day, most people are 'fast' as they sleep.

Intermittent fasting can be as easy as expanding it a little more quickly. Skip breakfast, eat your first meal at noon, and your last meal at 8 pm. Then you are fasting every day for 16 hours, technically speaking, and limiting your eating to an eating window of 8 hours. It is the most popular type of intermittent fasting, known as the method of 16/8.

In fact, it is quite easy to do intermittent fasting despite what you might think. Most people report that they feel better and that they have more energy in short. Hunger isn't usually a big concern, but it can be a problem at the beginning because the body won't eat for a long time.

During the fasting period, no food is allowed, but you can drink water, coffee, tea, and other non-caloric drinks. During the fasting period, some types of intermittent fasting allow small amounts of low-calorie food. It is generally allowed to take supplements while fasting, as long as there are no calories in them.

Why do we need to fast?

Indeed, for thousands of years, people have been fasting. It was done for religious reasons in other cases. Various religions mandate some form of fasting, including Islam, Christianity, and Buddhism. Also, people and other animals often fast instinctively when they are sick. Clearly, fasting is not 'unnatural,' and our bodies are very well equipped to handle long periods of non-eating.

When we don't eat for a while, all sorts of processes in the body change to allow our bodies to survive during a time of famine. It's about hormones, genes, and important processes of cellular repair. We get major reductions in blood sugar and insulin levels, as well as a dramatic rise in human growth hormone when fasted. Many people do intermittent fasting to lose weight, as it is a very simple and effective way to limit calories and burn fat. Others do this for the benefit of metabolic health, as different risk factors and health markers can be improved.

Intermittent fasting can help you live longer. Rhodes proves the lifespan can be extended as effectively as calories. There are also research signs that could help to protect against diseases such as cardiac disease, diabetes, cancer, Alzheimer's, etc. Others just like the convenience of intermittent fasting. It's an effective 'life hack' that makes life easier, while at the same time improving your health. The less food you need to plan, the easier your life will be.

Why is it so popular?

There are plenty of so-called benefits from intermittent fasting. Several studies suggest that intermittent fasting may result in weight loss, slowing the effects of aging, and even improving cardiovascular health.

As for the claims, your brain is helped by intermittent fasting? More studies suggest that intermittent fasting can improve cognition and even protect the brain from neurodegenerative diseases such as Alzheimer's. Experiencing hunger during periods of fasting, however, could have a significant impact on your ability to make decisions, think, and focus.

The loss of weight is another major draw. However, a study carried out in 2018 found that people who fasted intermittently for 50 weeks lost about an equal amount of weight as those who followed a traditional diet that limited their calories.
At the end of the day, while intermittent fasting may be trendy and enticing right now, it's not for everyone. It is not clear whether intermittent fasting is sustainable for long-term follow-up or those taking diabetes medication.
For example, intermittent fasting could put people at risk of developing deficiencies in nutrients. For some who have a history of eating disordered, intermittent fasting can lead to increased binge-eating or damage to their food relationship.

Persons that swear on it

Although intermittent fasting is perfect, big names have not stopped implementing their own intermittent raping routines.

For example, Dorsey, Twitter, and Square CEO fast every day and only eat between 6:30 pm. And nine a. And at 9 pm. He says that when he's not interrupted to eat, he can focus better. Dorsey said he would go on a weekend without eating from Friday night to Sunday night. It is an extreme example, for which Dorsey has been criticized (experts warn against extreme fasting over 24 hours).
'I found out that during these fasting times, I had much more to do because I was so focused, and it just seemed like I had much more time to think and work really at that moment,' Dorsey told Greenfield. It was helping him reach a whole new dimension.

Actor Jennifer Aniston makes an intermittent 16:8 fasting method, meaning she eats a daytime eight-hour window. 'I realized a major difference for 16 hours when I've been without solid food,' she said.

In addition, Kourtney Kardashian experimented some years ago with intermittent fasting and a very popular low-carb high-fat diet, ketogenic diet. 'I'm not going to eat after 7 pm. At night then I'd wait to eat until I'm around 10:30 am the next day after my morning workout. And 11 o'clock, 'she said. She'd just be drinking bone burnt broth, water, and green tea once a week for 24 hours.

Chris Hemsworth told that he was eating just by 12 pm And eight p.m. 'I consider my energy levels to be significantly increased and I found[that after you get over the initial shock of not eating[as regularly] in the first week or two weeks, your body is getting into another situation,' he said.

Chapter 1: Science behind intermittent fasting

In intermittent fasting studies, a recent systematic review has found a decrease in fat mass and both low-density. Lipoprotein (LDL) and triglyceride levels that showed improvements in cardiovascular health. Additional studies also suggest that these rapid schemes contribute to weight loss with potential effects on the metabolism and inflammation of glucose. These are also advantages shown by traditional diets for weight loss, suggesting that intermittent fasting can bring similar benefits.

Time-restricted eating, like other intermittent fasting regimens, is also associated with weight loss and may be important for optimal metabolic function. As we know, it is a diet limited by calories. Calorie restriction is currently the diet regimen that is most scientifically known to improve health. Improvements in cardiovascular disease risk factors, and type 2 diabetes, which include decreases in total cholesterol rates, blood triglycerides, blood pressure, carotid intima-media thickness, leptin, and fasting glucose, are the main advantages. Some people find the use of a calorie-deprived diet rare for an observable period of time incredibly difficult, and some find it impossible.

A 2015 systematic review of evidence from 40 different intermittent fasting studies in Molecular and Cellular Endocrinology reviewed. The researchers conclude that lowering body weight is useful. A 2017 study compared the effect of intermittent fasting on weight loss over one year and a standard calorie restriction diet. All dietary types were equally effective in weight loss. For other health markers, such as blood pressure or heart rate, there were no significant differences between the two groups. Much current research indicates that an efficient weight management technique may be intermittent fasting. It is unlikely that it will be more beneficial than the traditional restriction on calories, but some may find intermittent fasting easier.

In this chapter, you will know about what are the scientific effects of intermittent fasting on your brain, human growth hormone, insulin, ghrelin, and cholesterol level and how it helps you to fight cancer, to control your diabetes and inflammation.
So let's get a start.

1.1 Impacts on your brain health

Fasting has tremendous advantages in relation to a range of different functions of the brain. Perhaps the most important of these comes from a cycle of cellular cleaning called autophagy activation. All humans and mammals respond similarly when they are excessively depleted of calories, and the size of most of their major organs will decrease, that is to say, except for the brain and the testicles. It is said that this is to ensure the survival of these animals, and, on both counts, it makes a lot of sense.

What is autophagy activation?

Essentially, autophagy is where the body feeds itself. It sounds a bit scary, but it is actually one of the best things your body can train to do. It is the body's natural way of purifying itself from the inside out.

Autophagy plays a crucial role in regenerating, healing, and detoxifying the body itself. By activating this process, inflammation can be reduced, your brain functions optimized, and the aging process slowed. There are many types of research which prove that fasting promotes autophagy within the brain. It may enhance neuroplasticity, cognitive function, and brain structure. Intermittent fasting is an established means to activate autophagy.

History prevails

Though this fact may be unfamiliar to many, it is a highly researched subject, and the advantages of fasting have been known for a long time now. If you consider the way back when cavemen were around, and the food was a bit scarce during the winter months; if the normal functioning of the brain were to slow down on such occasions when food was limited, it would have made it almost impossible for those individuals to function and hunt for food. Nevertheless, it has been proven time and time again that during times of fasting, an enhanced cognitive function is attained. Other historical examples of this can be found in Ancient Greece, where fasting to enhance their mental agility was common practice for' The Great Thinkers.' Also, back then, it was highly regarded that hunger had a proven ability to sharpen one's mind and, respectively, improve cognitive ability.

Recent studies showing the effect of intermittent fasting on the brain

Professor Mark Mattson, the current Chief of Neuroscience Laboratory at The Johns Hopkins University's National Institute on Ageing and Professor of Neuroscience, gave a TEDx talk on the subject of fasting and its effects on the brain. Studies he published found that fasting triggered significant neurochemical changes in the brains of test subjects, leading to an increase in cognitive function and tolerance to stressful stimuli. These experiments also revealed a caloric restriction that decreased inflammation in the brain and increased neurotrophic factors such as neuron development and growth (which help with learning and memory). Professor Mattson also documented studies indicating fasting poses a brain challenge. The brain reacts to this task by modifying pathways for reaction to help it cope with stress. Interestingly, Professor Mattson outlined the reaction of the brain to intermittent fasting as being the same reaction that regular exercise requires. These behaviors affect the increased production of protein in the brain, which then facilitates neuronal growth and communication, and reinforces synapses.

Both of the practices also stimulate the production of nerve cells in the hippocampus, stimulate the production of ketones ('petrol' for neurons) and increase the number of mitochondria within the neurons, which in turn helps the neurons maintain their connections. All this has the net effect of improving memory and enhancing the learning capacity. He also said there were some signs that 'intermittent fasting improves nerve cells' ability to repair DNA.' If this is the case, focusing on preventive measures and possible treatment problems such as Dystonia and Dementia may be a good topic for research. In addition, some work that has been in this space has already shown positive results, according to Professor Mattson.

One aspect of the study that is especially interesting to note is that benefits were not attributed to a generally caloric restriction but to limited deliberate intermittent fasting times. All signs suggest that intermittent fasting not only has positive effects on your body, such as weight loss and risk factors enhancement with respect to heart disease, diabetes, and the like; it has an extremely positive impact on your brain, allowing increased focus and memory retention rates.

In fact, intermittent fasting can lead to improvements in memory and learning, as well as increasing greater brain resilience to conditions such as Dystonia and Dementia.

1.2 Boosts human growth hormones

HGH is a pituitary gland hormone that plays an important role in children's and adolescents' development. This hormone is also essential for adults, as a deficiency of HGH can lead to higher levels of body fat, lower lean body mass, and lower bone mass. HGH work starts by passing through the bloodstream and becoming metabolized in the liver. HGH is then converted into several other growth factors, the most important of which is the growth factor that resembles insulin. HGH, along with cortisol and adrenaline, is typically secreted just before waking up. Those hormones send signals to the body to increase glucose availability. Since HGH levels decrease with age, people seeking to adopt a healthier lifestyle may have essential health benefits.

If you fast, the human growth hormone, or somatotropin, increases. In normal circumstances, HGH stimulates lean muscle production and storage, both glycogen and fat. However, the increased hormone levels stimulate the breakdown of fatty tissue if you fast.

How does it work?

The increase in HGH during fasting helps preserve your stores of muscle tissue and glycogen while instead using your stores of fat. This degradation of fat, known as lipolysis, releases free fatty acids and glycerol, which are then metabolized for energy production. According to Madelon Buijs, a researcher at the Netherlands' Leiden University Medical Center, rates of HGH, which is released by the pituitary gland, increase significantly within 13 hours of a fast start.

Blood levels

In cases where there is a lack of HGH during fasting, muscle protein loss increases by around 50 percent. Besides fasting, exercise and stress can also raise rates of HGH. They also undergo a lot of variations during the day, as your pituitary gland releases the hormone in bursts. Random measurement of HGH is not very useful, in comparison to tracking it over time. What's more, morning rates will be higher.

Obesity

Insulin controls glucose metabolism for energy in non-fasting individuals, but HGH is predominant during times of fasting. Nevertheless, in obese individuals, lipolysis may be blunted during fasting periods due to various causes, which may be their lower levels of HGH. This effect may cause obese people to maintain adipose tissue. The lower HGH may, however, also protect them from the effects of excessively high levels of free fatty acids, which may be harmful to cells.

Benefits of high HGH

Higher levels of HGH contribute to loss of body fat, increase muscle mass, decrease the effects of aging on the skin, increase bone density, reinforce immunity, reverse cognitive decline, stimulate red blood cell production and decrease the risk of cardiovascular disease, according to 'Human Biochemistry and Disease.'

1.3 Improves insulin, ghrelin & cholesterol level

Understanding the role insulin plays is one of the major keys to understanding intermittent fasting.
Insulin, the hormone that controls blood sugar, is formed in the pancreas and released into the bloodstream as a reaction to food. Insulin is released, which causes the body to store energy as fat. Insulin produces fat, so the more insulin you make, the fat you store. The periods during intermittent fasting when you are not eating, give the body time to lower insulin levels, which reverses the process of fat storage. The process goes in reverse when the insulin levels drop, and you lose fat.

There are two other hormones at work too, ghrelin and leptin. Ghrelin is the hormone of appetite, which shows you when you're hungry. Some data suggest that ghrelin can diminish with intermittent fasting. There are also some data that say leptin, which is the satiety hormone, is on the increase. That's the one that says,' Oh, I'm finished.' With more leptin and less ghrelin, people will feel better and less hungry, which can result in fewer calories being eaten and weight loss as a result.

What benefits do you have?

People who fast may experience improved heart and brain functions due to reduced insulin, as well as weight loss. Think of your amount of insulin as the first domino in the entire body chain of what can happen with intermittent fasting. If you have high levels of insulin, this can lead to obesity, diabetes, high blood pressure, and high triglycerides. Together, those things are called metabolic syndrome, which raises cardiovascular disease risk. So, if your insulin level decreases, you'll probably lose weight, and your cholesterol, blood sugar, and blood pressure will improve.

Cholesterol drop may also decrease the inflammation caused by metabolic syndrome, namely plaque buildup in the arteries and cardiovascular inflammation in general. These improvements can also reduce people's risk of cardiovascular disease.

Even in the situation of weight loss, this cycle will happen. Some people may be on a strict regimen on an intermittent basis and fast. This effect is actually more common to what they consume than when they feed. When it comes to the brain, some data showed that lower levels of insulin could also minimize the damage in a person's brain cells, called neurons, which could theoretically reduce the risk of Parkinson's and Alzheimer's disease.

If there is less neuronal dysfunction, these conditions could possibly result in less risk. But that is still theoretical only. For example, the risk of Alzheimer's has been shown to be considerably higher in people with metabolic syndrome.

1.4 Helps to fight cancer

Some recent research suggests that fasting helps fight cancer by reducing insulin resistance and inflammatory rates. Intermittent fasting can also reverse the effects of chronic conditions like obesity and type 2 diabetes, which is both cancer risk factors.
Scientists also assume that, while protecting other cells, fasting will make cancer cells more receptive to chemotherapy. Fasting may also improve the immune system to help fight already established cancer. Some study has shown conditions such as obesity, and type 2 diabetes is cancer risk factors. Both are associated with a higher risk of multiple cancer types and lower rates of survival.

A case study from 2017 examined the effect of short-term fasting on type 2 diabetes. The study attendee fasted two to three times a week for 24 hours. The participant had a 17.8 percent weight loss and an 11 percent reduction in waist size following four months of fasting. After two months of this fasting pattern, they also no longer needed insulin treatment.

Improving the quality of life during chemotherapy

Many researchers believe that fasting enhances people's response to chemotherapy because it does the following:
1. Promotes cellular regeneration protects the blood from the harmful effects of chemotherapy
2. Reduces the impact of side effects such as weakness, headaches, and cramps.

A study found that fasting can improve the quality of life in people undergoing breast chemotherapy. The research used a 60-hour fasting period beginning 36 hours prior to the initiation of chemotherapy.

The results show that participants who were fasting during chemotherapy reported higher tolerance to chemotherapy, fewer side effects associated with chemotherapy, and higher levels of energy compared to those who did not fast.

Boosting the immune system to fight cancer

A 2014 study looked at whether fasting in mice stem cells has any cancer-fighting results. Stem cells are important because of their capacity to regenerate. The researchers revealed that 2-4 day fasting would protect stem cells from the negative effects of chemotherapy on the immune system. Fasting also stimulates immune system stem cells to rebuild and repair itself. This study shows that fasting not only decreases cell damage but replenishes white blood cells as well as replaces damaged ones.
White blood cells combat infection and can kill disease-causing cells. When the levels of white blood cells decrease as a result of chemotherapy, this will negatively affect the immune system. Which means the body is having a more difficult time battling infections. Through fasting, the number of white blood cells within the body reduces. Nevertheless, white blood cell levels increase when the fasting period ends, and the body receives food.

1.5 Reduces inflammation

Intermittent fasting and diets linked to it have a moment. And there may be some good reasons for extending their fame by 15 minutes. A new study concluded that intermittent fasting reduces inflammation, a condition that could lead to various diseases such as diabetes, multiple sclerosis, and inflammatory bowel syndrome. The drop, the study found, was due to a decrease in blood cells the cause inflammation— called 'monocytes.'

Scientists also said that the monocytes in the blood were less reactive than those in humans, and mice were not on an intermittent fasting diet. The reason for the difference may not be so much that it's safe to starve yourself to death as all the others eat too much. People eat all the time, especially in the Western world, and this is a relatively recent phenomenon in human evolution. Inflammation is a useful tool through which our bodies combat infections.

Yet, the volume of inflammation-causing cells that we usually have today may be more of an overeating option than a requirement. The findings from the study answer how that diet-inflammation connection works. But the lessons that eating less can reduce the inflammation and related problems aren't new.

Chapter 2: Why women should do intermittent fasting?

Intermittent fasting is becoming one of the most popular ways of weight loss and improving your health. It is no wonder: fasting works really well and produces incredible results for a lot of people. The advantages also go beyond weight loss: fasting can reduce inflammation, slow aging, and give you a stronger brain.

The other good thing about intermittent fasting is that it's beautifully simple: in a nutshell, you just eat 12-18 hours a day without food, and then in the remaining hours, eat all of your meals. However, if you have been following health and nutrition for a while, you may have heard that it is not great for women to be fasting. There's some irony there: while some women feel amazing when they're fasting, some run into trouble with their hormones in particular.

In this chapter, we will only discuss the benefits for the women that intermittent fasting actually provides. Those benefits are explained as below:

2.1 Healthier way to lose weight

If any woman wants to lose weight, but can't keep up with the hectic diet plans. Then, adopting intermittent fasting is the best and easiest way to lose weight. It's an eating pattern that's become popular among people seeking weight loss. It doesn't restrict your food choices or intake, unlike diets and other weight-loss programs. Instead, when you eat, all that matters is.

Firstly, it helps you lose your fats more effectively. Intermittent fasting will make the metabolism more energy-efficient at burning body fat. People who fasted intermittently lost more fat than people who continued a low-calorie diet.

How it helps you to lose weight?

Several studies show intermittent fasting can accelerate weight loss through multiple mechanisms.
Intermittent fasting triggers a perfect storm of changes in metabolism to deal with weight loss and fat reduction. How's it working out?

Reduces calories:

If you're a snacker or have a tendency to grab food on the go, you might eat more calories than your body needs–and that's going to show up on the scale. Generally speaking, you tend to eat less if you limit the amount of time you will eat during the day.

Kickstarts ketosis:

Intermittent fasting will speed up ketosis and accelerate weight loss when combined with ketogenic diets. The keto diet is intended to kick-start ketosis, which is very high in fats but low in carbs.

Ketosis is a metabolic state, which forces your body to burn fat instead of carbs for fuel. This happens when your body is deprived of glucose, which is its main energy source. The combination of intermittent fasting with the keto diet can help your body get into ketosis more quickly to maximize results. It can also reduce some of the side effects that often occur when this diet starts, including keto flu, which is characterized by nausea, headaches, and tiredness.

Intermittent fasting is a precursor to ketosis in the fat-burning process. Via their glucose stores (aka carbohydrates), your body burns for energy during your fast. Then, you begin to burn fat for fuel. Eat a ketogenic diet during fasting times, to optimize weight loss.

Down insulin levels:

Intermittent fasting has two effects on insulin. Next, the body becomes more insulin reactive, which can help prevent weight gain and reduce your diabetes risk. Second, fasting reduces your insulin levels, which can cause the body to start burning stored fat instead of glucose.

Boosts metabolism:

Intermediate fasting reprogrammed metabolic ways to extract more energy from food. Fasting also increases your adrenaline and noradrenaline levels, hormones that allow the body to release more stored power during a quick time. The restful metabolism increases the body's calories all day, even while you rest.

Multiple studies show weight loss accelerated by intermittent fasting. On average, participants shed 10 pounds in a 2015 review pooling 40 different studies over a 10-week period. Another smaller study of 16 obese adults after an irregular 'alternate day' fasting regimen resulted in a loss of up to 13 pounds over eight weeks.

2.2 May extend your life-span

Other than weight loss, another obvious benefit of intermittent fasting has come to the fore. A recent study indicates that intermittent fasting can increase a person's life span. Cardiac catheterization is a method used to identify certain cardiovascular problems and to treat them. Study scientists believe that intermittent fasting may produce positive health outcomes for cardiac catheterization patients. You will live longer and are less likely to get a heart failure diagnosis.

What recent research says?

A new study conducted by Harvard researchers has now shown how fasting can increase lifespan, slow aging, and improve health by altering mitochondrial network activity within our cells. While previous work has shown how intermittent fasting can slow aging, we are only beginning to understand the biology that underlies it. In our cells, mitochondria are a bit like tiny power plants.

A team of researchers last year successfully demonstrated how mitochondria are central to cell aging. Harvard's new research shows how evolving types of mitochondrial networks can affect longevity and lifespan, but more importantly, the study reveals how fasting manipulates those mitochondrial networks in order to keep them in a 'youthful' state. Within cells, mitochondrial networks generally differentiate between two states: fused and fragmented.

A team of researchers last year successfully demonstrated how mitochondria are fundamental to cell aging. Harvard's new research shows how changing forms of mitochondrial networks can affect longevity and lifespan, but more importantly, the study illustrates how fasting manipulates those mitochondrial networks in order to keep them in a 'youthful' condition.

Within cells, mitochondrial networks usually vary between two states: fused and broken. The study found that restricted diets facilitate homeostasis in mitochondrial networks allowing healthy plasticity between these fused and fragmented states. The study also found that intermittent fasting improves mitochondrial communication with peroxisomes, a form of organelle that can increase oxidized fatty acid. In experiments conducted in the study, the women's lifespan was increased by simply preserving homeostasis of the mitochondrial network through dietary intervention. These results help to shed some light on how fasting can increase longevity and encourage healthy aging of women as well as men.

Low-energy treatments, including dietary restriction and intermittent fasting have been shown historically to promote healthy aging. Knowing why that is the case is a crucial step towards being able to maximize the benefits therapeutically. New findings open up new avenues in the search for therapeutic strategies that will reduce our chance of developing age-related diseases as we grow older.

2.3 Boost your immune system

Apart from raising your life span intermittent fasting, the immune system also enhances. In short, intermittent fasting reduces white blood cell counts, which activates stem-cell-based regeneration of new immune system cells, which not only enhances your immunity but also plays a role in longevity.

The fasting method allows the body to concentrate more of your energy and focus on the successful immune response cycle. You are fasting while drinking water, and cleaning drinks flush the digestive system and reduces the number of natural microorganisms in the gut. The count of microorganisms is typically regulated by the immune system. So this helps the immune system to transfer resources to other places of greater importance.

Intermittent fasting is a powerful immune system regulator because it regulates the number of inflammatory cytokines released into the body. Two major Interleukin-6 cytokines and the Alpha tumor necrosis factor facilitate an inflammatory response in the body. Studies have shown that fasting reduces those inflammatory mediators ' release. Modulation of the immune system, which provides intermittent fasting, can also be helpful if you have moderate to severe allergies.

How can three days intermittent fasting can reset your immune system?

Ladies! Want to boost your immune system in the first place, so you don't even catch that cold? Forget the large amounts of vitamin C or drastic changes in lifestyle; it turns out that the old adage of starving a cold can be scientifically sound advice indeed. That's according to a study that says fasting resets immune systems for two to four days, benefiting everyone from healthy women to chemotherapy women.

Research in both mice and humans have shown that prolonged fasting times have significantly reduced white blood cell counts, according to a review. It leads to a transition in the signaling pathways of HSCs or hematopoietic stem cells, creating new blood and immune systems.

One of the writers of the study, Valter Longo, said, 'When you're hungry, the system is trying to save energy, and one of the things it can do to save energy is to recycle a lot of unnecessary immune cells, especially those that can be damaged.'
This can be particularly beneficial for elderly women and those with autoimmune disorders that are more susceptible to disease and disease.

2.4 Maintain a more youthful appearance

Most people go to a beauty salon or plastic surgeon in order to look better and have a youthful appearance. We don't mind recruiting a lot of money to get rid of their face's wrinkles. Exercise helps make you look young, and so does sleep. And getting older is a natural law that needs to be observed. But do you know why you look younger with intermittent fasting.

Currently no need to spend too much money on beauty services or costly beauty products for those who want to stay young because other than boosting your immune system and making you lose your weight in a healthier way, it also makes you look younger. Shocked?

Now you think that how it is possible to look younger by just fasting. Factly and scientifically, it is true that through intermittent fasting, your youthful appearance can be maintained.

There's more evidence that the weight loss and anti-aging advantages of this form of intermittent fasting. Eating really lightly will actually make you prevent illnesses and keep those wrinkles at bay.

People who ate a special low-calorie diet for five days in a month lost weight had lower cholesterol rates, lower blood pressure, and lower body fat measurements, according to new studies. Dieters take off about five pounds on a diet after three months on average and tend to have improved blood sugar control, which reduces their risk of diabetes. It has also been found that they have fewer signs of inflammation, which is a significant contributor to cancer, heart disease, and obesity.

Intermittent fasting will keep your body healthier, prolong your lifespan, and improve your overall health. As you have already read: Harvard researchers found that temporarily restricting diet maintains the mitochondria–an important part of the cell for health aging–in homeostasis, which in turn helps improve lifespan.

Some studies have shown that intermittent fasting has no benefit over normal dietary restrictions, but animal studies have found it to be related to longer life spans. Newcastle University research last year verified the crucial role that mitochondria plays in the aging of human cells, and hence the aging of our bodies.

Breaks down carbohydrates and fatty acids and gives the cell strength. They are often referred to as our cell's" powerhouses' for this reason. The researchers at Newcastle University noticed that cells seemed younger without their aged mitochondria. This profound knowledge of how fasting operates at the cellular level could be a key to finding treatments that could be useful for extending life expectancies and keeping the body younger.

What happens to your body when we apply intermittent fasting?

Fasting in our body, particularly in the digestive tract, can reduce or temporarily stop the physiological processes or metabolism. Termination of the metabolic process brings with it four sets of processes that have a major health effect.

1. Limit the amount of food coming into the digestive tract.
2. Lowered digestive system pressure.
3. All endotoxins (toxins from the body itself) and exotoxins (toxins from outside the body) also decrease with the decrease in work intensity.
4. Reducing the ingredients that need to be digested will also not cause our bodies to release large-scale hormones and digestive enzymes.

Imagine that if we don't fast? All foods entering the body have to be digested to be certain. They would probably be pushing our digestive organs to work harder.

Intermittent fasting gives you a youthful feel. The so-called youth, already a common concept among experts, is simply an uncontrolled cycle of premature aging. Our body begins to age as early as 25 years old even though we don't notice it.

2.5 Cause of autophagy

Forget healing water and food detox. There's probably anything right with drinking your weight in liquid kale; it's not going to flush out contaminants any faster than eating actual food, you know.

The good news: The body cleanses itself in a little-known way, and it's a method that you can optimize. You just have to practice a little self-cannibalism.
What? How is it possible? It can be possible through intermittent fasting, also by ketogenic diet, and also by exercising.

What does it mean?

The Greek word derives from auto (self) and phagein (eat). Thus the word literally means eating yourself. Essentially, this is the body's process to get rid of all the broken down, old cell machinery (organelles, proteins, and cell membranes) when there is not enough capacity to support it any longer. The degradation and recycling of cellular components is a supervised, orderly process.

Apoptosis, also known as programmed cell death, is a related, better-known process. Cells happened to die after a certain number of divisions. While this may at first sound like a macabre, realize that this process is essential to maintaining good health.
Cells get old and junky. It's better to have them programmed to die when their useful lives are completed. It really sounds cruel, but it's life. This is the apoptosis process, where cells are predestined to die after some time. It is like leasing an automobile. You get rid of the car after a certain amount of time, whether it is still running or not.

Then you get yourself a new car. You need not worry about breaking it down at the worst possible time.

What benefits do women have of autophagy?

There is some evidence to suggest that autophagy plays a role, among other benefits, in reducing inflammation and boosting immunity. Researchers found in one 2012 study that autophagy protected from:

1. Cancer
2. Disorders Neurodegenerative
3. Illnesses
4. Inflammatory illnesses
5. Age
6. Insulin resistance

Another study that year showed how harmful a lack of autophagy could be. Researchers found weight gain, lethargy, higher cholesterol, and impaired brain function were caused by the removal of the autophagy gene.

In short, autophagy makes us more efficient machines to eliminate deficiencies, stop cancerous growth, and stop metabolic dysfunction such as obesity and diabetes.

How to kick start autophagy?

'How can I feed myself, then?' It's probably a question you've never asked, but we're going to tell you why. Autophagy is a reaction to stress, so you're going to want your body to drum up a little bit of extra self-cannibalism through some hardship.

That hardship is to do intermittent fasting.

Deprivation of nutrients is the key activator of autophagy. Recall that insulin is kind of the opposite hormone to glucagon. It's like the game that we played as children -'opposite day.' If insulin goes up, then glucagon will go down. If insulin falls, glucagon will rise. The insulin goes up as we eat, and the glucagon goes down. When we don't eat (fast), insulin will go down, and glucagon will go up. That glucagon increase stimulates the autophagy process. Fasting (raises glucagon) actually provides the biggest known boost to autophagy.

Fasting is indeed far more beneficial than simply stimulating autophagy. They're doing two good things. We're clearing out all our old, junky proteins and cellular parts by stimulating autophagy. Simultaneously, fasting also stimulates growth hormone, which tells our body to start producing some new snazzy body parts. We are really giving the whole renovation to our bodies.

Before you can put in new stuff, you must get rid of the old stuff. Think of having your kitchen renovated. If you have old lime green cabinets sitting around in the 1970s style, you need to junk them before you put some new ones in. So, the destruction process (removal) is just as important as the creation process. If you were simply trying to put the old cabinets in without taking them out, it wouldn't look so hot. So intermittent fasting may reverse the aging process by getting rid of old cellular junk and replacing it with new parts.

2.6 Increased your ketones

Maybe it's not surprising that many also adopt an intermittent fasting keto diet. You may be one of those people. That makes sense— keto and intermittent fasting both have much in common. Keto works much the same way intermittent fasting does.
And, in fact, sticking to a low-carbohydrate or ketogenic diet can actually make intermittent fasting much, much easier to practice. The combination of keto with intermittent fasting will offer the body some quite remarkable benefits.

Overview of ketosis

Ketosis is a metabolic condition characterized by ketones inside the blood. This happens when the body faces a 'challenge' of low blood sugar and reduced glycogen stores, which initiates a cascade of hormones signaling the body to start breaking down fat stores and release fatty acids into the circulation.

Such fatty acids are transferred to the liver once in circulation and used in the development of ketones— a process called ketogenesis. The liver, in particular, develops a ketone body called acetoacetate (AcAc), the bulk of which is converted into beta-hydroxybutyrate (BHB).

What is ketosis for?

Most of us know that consuming carbohydrates as well as fat will create energy for our bodies. One of the major energy sources for humans and animals is glucose— which we acquire primarily through consuming dietary carbohydrates: bread, nuts, grains, legumes, starches, and sugars. One reason we control blood sugar is the conversion of carbohydrates into glucose. Lots of body tissues use glucose as a fuel— and some don't use anything else (for example, some eye cells and red blood cells).

We can store glucose in our muscles and liver as glycogen— long chains of glucose, in addition to glucose in the blood. We use glycogen in conditions where blood glucose starts running low, like in long-term exercise. Fat and lipids are also a great source of energy because we have a lot of it! Even the skinniest among us have ample body fat to last long.

Ketosis is intended to provide fuel when other energy sources (mainly glucose) are running low. This was (and perhaps still is) a survival mechanism that allowed species to live under conditions where food supplies were small. In order to maintain high energy levels and cognitive function, the liver generates ketones to support the brain and body as a metabolic fuel.

Unlike fatty acids, ketones can cross the blood-brain barrier, which separates the brain from our circulation. In this way, when glucose is small, the brain can have an energy source. Up to 60 percent of brain energy can come from ketone body metabolism during 'starvation.'

While in our modern time's ketosis is not really required for 'survival,' this 'special' metabolic state probably has some benefits. In this post, we will be speaking factly about endogenous ketosis, because it is better linked to intermittent fasting.

Fasting research has shown that this lifestyle practice can have a multitude of health benefits— some of which are similar to ketosis-induced ones. That makes sense; fasting contributes to the development of ketones. Let's look at how that is going to happen.

Ketones production due to intermittent fasting

Each time we eat, it causes a metabolic response. The metabolic reaction will include an increase in blood glucose (of varying degrees) and insulin if the meal includes carbohydrates. The pancreas releases insulin to facilitate blood glucose absorption into our skeletal muscles.

Once insulin is released, excess energy stored as glycogen or adipose tissue is indicated for the body. The primary place of storage is the muscle of the liver and the skeleton. Along with upregulating energy storage processes, insulin inhibits others—especially those that release fat from our stored adipose tissue deposits. Because no food enters, blood glucose and insulin levels begin to drop throughout fasting. The body will start burning fat after a certain period of time and will generate ketones. How long will it take for this?

The concentrations of ketones in the body are around 0.1-0.5mM after a single overnight high, meaning you will be just below the 'threshold' for ketosis. The ketones will hit 1-2mM after 48 hours of fasting. Five days of fasting will increase ketone levels to about 7-8mM.[19] Fat burning and ketone production are the main effects of intermittent fasting
And now, you are thinking about the benefits of ketone levels. Actually, they really have positive effects on your body. That you really need to learn.

Benefits you have from this?

They have the following positive effects in your body:
1. It helps your body to lose weight.

2. It also helps your body to control your cholesterol and diabetes.
3. It also helps in the treatment of certain epilepsy.

In short, all of these benefits can be gained when you do intermittent fasting.

2.7 Reduce inflammations

Experts say people are unnecessarily inflamed because they eat too much and eat too often. And this inflammation is one way in which the body fights infection, but if there is too much inflammation that can lead to many diseases. Recent research indicates that intermittent fasting in women, in particular, can reduce inflammation in your body.

How can intermittent fasting fight inflammation?

Intermittent fasting is a general term for a time in which you limit or do not consume food intake at all. Why would anybody need to put themselves through times of hunger? Okay, studies have shown that intermittent fasting could bring down inflammation markers significantly. In reality, research shows a few interesting ways in which intermittent fasting calms down various types of inflammation:

Brain inflammation

Problems with mental health such as anxiety, depression, and brain fog are on the rise, and studies show that IF enhances brain function and mood, having a kind of antidepressant impact. Neurological conditions such as Alzheimer's and Parkinson's are known as neuroinflammatory diseases, as well as mood disorders such as depression and anxiety, and IF also looks positive for these. Many studies have shown that IF can actually protect neurons from genetic and epigenetic stress factors, suggesting that brain aging can be basically slowed down!

Lung inflammation

For one study, it was shown that fasting every other day decreases the symptoms of asthma and signs of oxidative stress and inflammation.

Hormone signaling inflammation

Intermittent fasting reduces insulin resistance, a metabolic problem affecting a whopping 50 percent of American adults! It also increases the development of beneficial enzymes that improve the capacity of your body to respond to stress and fight chronic diseases such as diabetes.

Chronic pain inflammation

Intermittent fasting enhances something called neuroplasticity — the brain's ability to form and reorganize synaptic connections in response to new information — which researchers are studying for the function it may play in chronic pain management.

Gut inflammation

IF can be a problem for inflammatory intestines such as pain in the stomach, IBS, colitis, vomiting, and nausea. Evidence also demonstrates the benefits of gut health from fasting therapy.

Heart inflammation

Over addition, IF has been shown to reduce the risk of cardiovascular disease due to its ability to increase healthy HDL cholesterol and reduce triglycerides and blood pressure.

I hope now you are truly aware of the importance and benefits of intermittent fasting. In the next chapter, you will learn about how a woman should do intermittent fasting. Normally, there are many different ways of intermittent fasting; it's all up to you what method is suitable to you and your body.

Chapter 3: How women should do intermittent fasting?

In recent years, intermittent fasting has been very common. It is said to have caused a loss of weight, enhanced metabolic health, and likely longer life. Not surprisingly, given the popularity of intermittent fasting, several different types or methods were created. More than one way of implementing intermittent fasting is feasible, although different methods produce different results. I also included most of the intermittent fasting strategies studied in this chapter in order to select the approach that is appropriate for you.

The intermittent fasting experience of each person is unique, and different types are appropriate for different people. We discuss the investigations behind the most popular types of intermittent fasting in this chapter and provide tips on how to keep this type of diet. Read about all the approaches and pick the fasting schedule that suits your goals and type of body.

3.1 The 5:2 intermittent fasting

Sometimes known as 'The 5:2 Fast DietTM' or 'The Easy Diet' or 'Intermittent Fasting' is the 5:2 diet. It is based on the underlying principle of eating 'normally' for five days out of 7 (not being overly calorie-conscious and not avoiding other foods) and then 'fasting' for the other two days out of 7.

Yet, 'fasting' doesn't mean you're doing anything. This means eating about a fifth of your daily calorie intake in the 5:2 diet. Men and women have different daily calorie levels, which are recommended. On a fasting day, a woman on the 5:2 diet should consume about 500 calories in total, and a man should eat about 600 calories.

The 500 or 600 calories can be consumed as snacks, or as one or two meals throughout the day. And the two days of fasting needn't be identical-they could be a Tuesday and Friday, for example.

Better foods to eat on a 'fasting' day are supposed to be foods high in protein and fiber that help to fill you up more-so items like seafood, meat, and vegetables.

There are a number of people endorsing the 5:2 diet and promoting it. These involve Michael Mosley, who was originally trained as a doctor, then became a BBC producer and presenter. Mr. Mosley adopted the 5:2 diet for the first time during the 2012 BBC Horizon program.

It is a slightly misleading term for fasting. Unlike a true fast that involves eating nothing for a set amount of time, the goal of the 5:2 diet is to limit caloric intake to 25 percent on fasting days, or just one-quarter of a person's daily intake on the remaining days.

For example, a person who regularly eats around 2,000 calories per day on days of fasting will eat 500 calories. Importantly, fasting days aren't identical because giving the body the calories and nutrients it needs to thrive is important.

For example, by having their reduced-calorie days on Monday and Thursday or Wednesday and Saturday, people typically spread their fasting days out.

Instead of severely restricting the food a person may consume, the 5:2 diet focuses only on two days of the week on strict caloric restriction. This can help some people feel more satisfied with their diet, as they won't feel they're missing out on all the time.

Nevertheless, the five normal days of the 5:2 diet should still require a healthy diet. Loading up for five days on sugary or fried foods and then taking a slight break may not be as effective as sustaining a routine of healthy eating during the week.

What are the benefits?

The 5:2 diet can have several advantages, including:

Weight loss

Nutritionists call that a deficiency of calories. When someone correctly follows this, the 5:2 diet can be a simple, easy way to cut calories, which can help burn extra fat. Although there aren't many clear studies on the 5:2 diet, initial intermittent fasting studies seem encouraging.

An analysis in the Annual Nutrition Analysis indicated that a similar intermittent fasting diet in animal studies has resulted in a decrease in fat tissue and the cells that store fat.

A 2018 study and meta-analysis compared intermittent fasting to diets that limit basic calories. This study indicated that intermittent fasting is as effective when it comes to weight loss and enhancing metabolic health as calorie restriction.

Reducing the risk of type 2 diabetes

Initial studies also indicate a daily calorie diet can also help to reduce the risk of diabetes in some individuals.

Data from 2014 shows that in adults who were overweight or obese, both intermittent fasting diets and calorie-restriction diets helped reduce fasting insulin levels and insulin resistance. In order to confirm these results, the reviewers have called for more studies. This does not mean that intermittent fasting is a better diet, merely an equally effective option for people who find it difficult to eat under calorie restriction.

How to eat on fast days?

There is no better way to eat on days of intermittent fasting, as the body of each person will respond to fasting differently. The theory is that a person consumes only 25% of their normal calorie intake on fast days.

Many people may need to start the day with a little breakfast, for example, to get their body moving. For others, eating breakfast at once can make them feel more hungry all day long. Many women may want to wait for their first meal as long as possible.
Because of that, the meal plan will look slightly different for everyone. The main focus of the day is for a woman to reduce the calories they consume drastically.

If a person eats 2,000 calories per day on a regular basis, they can consume just 500 calories on the intermittent fast days. A woman who usually eats 1,800 calories a day on fast days can lower their consumption to 450 calories.

Foods to include

It is vital to keep the body happy by eating foods that are rich in nutrient-filled, such as fiber and protein, on fast days.

Vegetables and fiber

For people who are just starting out on the 5:2 diet, eating more vegetables will help them feel like they're not missing during a meal. Compared with animal products and grains, vegetables can be very low in calories.

Protein

Protein is essential for fast days to remain fresh. Without too much fat, people should focus on lean protein sources. In fast days, add small amounts of lean protein types,
Including whitefish lean animal cuts egg beans and lentils tofu. Importantly, people can avoid oil and fats by boiling, grilling, or roasting these foods instead of frying them.

Dark berries

While the majority of fruits are high in natural sugars, dark berries, such as blackberries and blueberries, will satisfy sweet cravings without adding many calories.

Other foods

a. Soup: It is a great tool for fast days because the added water and spices from the soup will make a person feel more satisfied without eating too many calories.
b. Water: Water is important every day, but it can help stretch the time between meals during the fast days and prevent a person from experiencing hunger pangs.
c. Coffee or tea: It is appropriate to have simple, unsweetened coffee and tea during the fast days. Some people, however, find

that coffee or tea stimulates their digestive system, which makes them feel hungry. Herbal tea is another choice and is a great way to increase the water intake of the person.

Food to avoid

To avoid extra calories or to use the daily calorie limit on foods with less nutritional advantages than some other, more nutrient-dense ones, a person may want to avoid the following fast-day foods:
Processed foods, usually refined and high in calories, such as bread and pasta, including cooking oils, animal fats, and cheese.

How to eat on regular days?

A person eats as they would normally, on regular days. It's important to note that these five daily days are not 'cheat days'. That's why keeping within the acceptable calorie limit and consuming a variety of nutritious foods is still beneficial.
A woman who eats plenty of fried, packaged, or unhealthy foods will probably notice fewer weight changes from fasting.

3.2 The 16/8 method

16:8 intermittent fasting is a popular type of fasting, also called the 16:8 diet or 16:8 program. People who follow this eating plan are going to fast 16 hours a day and consume all their calories over the remaining 8 hours. The 16:8 plan's potential advantages include weight loss and fat loss, as well as the prevention of type 2 diabetes and other disorders associated with obesity.

Learn more about the intermittent 16:8 fasting program, including how to do it, health benefits, and side effects.

What is 16/8 intermittent fasting?

16:8 intermittent fasting is a time-restricted type of fasting. This involves eating food during an8-hour period and refusing food, or fasting, every day for the remaining 16 hours.

Many people think this method works by promoting the circadian rhythm of the body, which is its inner clock. Many people who follow the 16:8 program abstain in the morning and evening from food. During the middle of the day, they prefer to eat their daily calories. There are no limits on the types or quantities of food a person can eat during the eight-hour window. Such versatility makes the strategy to be implemented relatively easily.

How to do it?

The best way to follow the 16:8 diet is to pick a 16-hour fasting period with the time a person spends sleeping. Several experts suggest stopping food consumption early in the evening, as, after this time, metabolism slows down. This is not feasible, however. Many people may not be able to eat up their dinner until 7 p.m. Or at a later date. Even so, it is best to avoid 2–3 hours of food before bedtime.

Users can choose one of the following feeding times across 8 hours:
1. 9 a.m. to 5 P.M.
2. 10:00 AM to 6 P.M.
3. Noon to 8 p.m.

Visitors will eat their meals and snacks at convenient times within this timeframe. Regular eating is important to prevent peaks and drops in blood sugar and to prevent excessive hunger.

Recommended foods and tips

While the intermittent 16:8 fasting program doesn't specify which foods to consume and avoid, concentrating on healthy eating and restricting or eliminating junk foods is beneficial. Too much unhealthy food intake can cause weight gain and lead to illness. Balanced intermittent fasting focuses primarily on: fruits and vegetables, beef, beans, lentils, tofu, nuts, berries, low-fat cottage cheese, and eggs healthy fats from olives, olive oil, coconuts, avocados, nuts, and seeds. Healthy fats and proteins can also play a part in satiety.

For those adopting the 16:8 intermittent fasting diet, beverages may play a part in satiety. Drinking water more often throughout the day will help to reduce calorie intake as people often confuse hunger thirst. The 16:8 diet plan calls for calorie-free drinks— like water and unsweetened tea and coffee— to drink during the 16 hour fasting period. To prevent dehydration, it is important to consume fluids regularly.

Health benefits

For decades scientists have been investigating intermittent fasting. The findings of the study are sometimes conflicting and inconclusive. Nonetheless, research on intermittent fasting, including 16:8 fasting, suggests that it could provide the following benefits:

Weight loss and fat loss

Eating over a set period can help people reduce the number of calories they consume. It can help to boost metabolism too. A study conducted in 2017 shows that intermittent fasting in men with obesity results in greater weight loss and fat loss than daily calorie restriction.

Two thousand sixteen research reports that women who practiced an eight-week 16:8 strategy during resistance training saw a reduction in fat mass. The participants retained throughout their muscle mass.

In comparison, a 2017 study found very little difference in weight loss between participants who practiced intermittent fasting–in the form of alternate-day fasting rather than 16:8 fasting –and those who decreased their overall calorie intake. The dropout rate among those in the intermittent fasting category was also very high.

Prevention of disease

Intermittent fasting proponents say that it can prevent many disorders and illnesses, including; type 2 diabetes heart conditions of certain cancers and neurodegenerative diseases.

Nonetheless, the researchers warn that more research is needed before accurate conclusions can be drawn. A 2018 study shows that an8-hour eating period will help reduce blood pressure in adults with obesity, in addition to weight loss.

Some studies report that intermittent fasting in people with prediabetes decreases fasting glucose by 3–6 percent, although it has no effect on healthy people. It may also decrease insulin fasting by 11–57 percent after intermittent fasting for 3 to 24 weeks. Time-limited fasting, such as the 16:8 process, can also support learning and memory and slow down brain-influencing diseases. A 2017 annual review states that animal research has been shown to reduce the risk of non-alcoholic fatty liver disease and cancer by this type of fasting.

An extended period of life

Animal studies say intermittent fasting can allow animals to live longer. For example, one study found that repeated fasting over the short term increased female mice's lifespan.

The National Institute for Aging points out that even after decades of research, scientists are still unable to understand why fasting can extend the life span. Consequently, they cannot guarantee this practice's long-term protection. Human studies in the region are minimal, and the potential benefits to human longevity from intermittent fasting are not yet understood.

Side effects and risks

16:8 intermittent fasting has certain risks and side effects associated with that. As a result, not everyone gets the plan right. Potential side effects and risks include:
Nausea, exhaustion, and fatigue in the early stages of the program overeating or eating unhealthy foods during the8-hour eating period due to excessive appetite heartburn or reflux is resulting from overeating.

Intermittent fasting may be less beneficial to women than men. Some animal research indicates intermittent fasting could have an adverse effect on female fertility. Women with disordered eating history may wish to avoid intermittent fasting.

The 16:8 program may not suit those with a history of depression and anxiety, either. Some research suggests that short-term calorie restriction may reduce depression, but chronic calorie restriction may have the opposite effect. To understand the implications of those results, further research is needed. 16:8 intermittent fasting is unacceptable for those women who are pregnant, lactating, or trying to conceive.

3.3 Eat, stop, eat method

There are numerous ways of doing intermittent fasting. The 5:2 diet, 12-hour fasts, 16-hour fasts, and 20-hour fasts, for example. While each strategy has its own share of benefits and risks, it does seem easier to adopt the Eat Stop Eat approach. Note, if you can follow a fasting strategy without changing your daily schedule drastically, you'll probably stick to it for longer durations. Simply put, a 'regular' uphill struggle should not be to adopt an ideal fasting process.

Intermittent fasting is practically everywhere-celebrities swear by its benefits, scientists explore new 'potential' benefits every other day, and health magazines often have it in the headlines.

Ironically, some experts in nutrition go so far as to say that IF's unparalleled success might actually harm it may credibility. We are afraid it could end up like any other fad. Their concern is understandable and reasonable to some degree. That said, there is enough evidence to support the benefits of intermittent fasting, at least if you are doing it for a short period of time.

Basic knowledge of this method

Eat Stop Eat is Fasting Expert Brad Pilon's brainchild. Brad was conducting research on the effects of short-term fasting during his graduate studies at the University of Guelph, Guelph Ontario, Canada. He used the research findings to formulate the book Eat Stop Eat.

Brad states that 24-hour fasting once or twice a week is one of the most effective ways of losing extra pounds. You will normally eat during the non-fasting days, but during the days of fasting, you must refrain from any hard food or calorie-containing drink. This way, you'll build a calorie deficit that can help you lose weight over time.

Benefits of Eat, stop, eat method

When you search Google for Eat Stop Eat analysis, you'll find hundreds of positive reviews from people who've done it. For one such study, a blogger reports that after a 4-week struggle, they lost four kilos/9 pounds. While you may lose more (or less) weight with this strategy, what's sure is that you'll shed a few pounds.

Since Eat Stop Eat is an intermittent fasting process, you should expect a variety of other benefits such as the lower risk of type 2 diabetes, improved heart health, decreased brain inflammation, and lower cancer risk. One of Eat Stop Eat's key benefits is that it doesn't allow you to die of starvation each day.

You can eat anything you want, 5 or 6 days a week. You have to swift for 24 hours during the days of fasting. You can fast once to twice a week, depending on your schedule and lifestyle. Such versatile scheduling allows you to enjoy your party, have breakfast with your loved ones, or go with your sweetheart on a dinner date.

Why might it be a perfect choice for newbies?

You don't have to fast every day, which may affect your daily schedule in some cases. You would certainly not want your children to miss breakfast just because you are fasting. Compared with other IF approaches such as the 5:2 diet, 16-hour fasts, and 20-hour fasts, sticking to Eat Stop Eat is better for some. Some weekend days, you may choose to fast when you can engage in activities to relieve yourself from cravings.

Eat Stop Eat can sound similar to the 5:2 diet for a newbie. There is, however, a significant difference between these two methods. The 5:2 diet allows for the consumption of about 500 calories during the days of fasting, but with Eat Stop Eat, you must refrain from eating for a whole 24-hour cycle.

It seems impossible to eat nothing for 24 hours, right? Though, remember to eat 500 calories (when fasting) will cause appetite. On the other hand, intaking nothing for 24 hours effectively suppresses malnutrition.

Should you try this?

Now, the million-dollar question comes here, and the answer is hell, yes!

The method to Eat Stop Eat is easy to follow, flexible and will suit your schedule unless you're super busy. You can fast on weekend days, even if you're super busy. This way, you can get all the advantages you'd get from other sporadic forms of fasting.

Eat Stop Eat isn't just a pure fasting process. Instead, it is a philosophy focussing on intermittent feeding breaks. Nonetheless, it's important to know your needs, goals, and skill before you opt for Eat Stop Eat or any other fasting process.

3.4 Alternate-day intermittent fasting

Another way to do intermittent fasting is to do alternate-day fasting. On that diet, you fast every other day, but on non-fasting days, eat whatever you want. However, the most common version of this diet involves 'adjusted' fasting, where you can consume 500 calories on a fasting day. Alternate-day fasting is a very powerful tool for weight loss and can help reduce the risk of heart disease and type 2 diabetes.
Detailed information on alternate-day fasting is available here.

How to do this type of intermittent fasting?

Alternate-day fasting (ADF) is a fasting method that is intermittent.

The basic idea is that one day you run and the next day you eat what you want. This way, you just have to limit what you eat half the time. You're allowed to drink as many calorie-free drinks as you like on Fasting days. Examples include beer, tea, and unsweetened coffee.

When you follow a modified ADF plan, you'll also be allowed to eat around 500 calories on days of fasting, or 20–25% of your energy needs.

The weight loss benefits seem to be the same irrespective of whether intermittent fasting-day calorie intake at lunch, dinner, or as small meals throughout the day. Studies show that many people find alternate-day fasting much easier to adhere to than traditional, daily calorie restrictions. This is considered much more manageable on fasting days than doing complete fasts, but it is just as successful.

The terms 'alternate-day fasting' or 'ADF' generally apply to the adapted method for fasting days with around 500 calories.

Alternate-day fasting and weight loss

For weight loss, ADF is very powerful. Studies of overweight and obese adults show that in 2–12 weeks, you can lose 3-8 percent of your body weight. Interestingly, for weight loss among middle-aged people, ADF seems to be particularly effective. Research has shown that ADF and the daily calorie restriction in obese individuals are similarly effective in reducing unhealthy belly fat and inflammatory markers.

Nonetheless, a review study conducted in 2016 found that ADF may be preferable to normal diets for calorie restriction, as it is easier to stick to, result in greater fat loss and retain more muscle mass. In fact, combining ADF with endurance exercise will cause weight loss twice as much as ADF alone. As for the nature of the food, ADF tends to be equally effective, whether it is achieved with a high-fat or low-fat diet.

Alternate-day fasting and hunger

ADF's impacts on hunger are rather incongruous. Several studies show that, in the end, hunger goes down on days of fasting, while others claim that hunger remains the same.

Evidence nevertheless agrees that adjusted ADF on fasting days with 500 calories is much more tolerable than absolute fasts on fasting days. One study comparing ADF to calorie restriction found that ADF induced somewhat more beneficial shifts in the leptin satiety hormone and the ghrelin hunger hormone.

Likewise, animal studies have shown that improved ADF has led to lower concentrations of hunger hormones and increased levels of satiety hormones relative to other diets.
This aspect that wants to be considered is compensatory hunger, a common drawback to typical daily calorie restrictions.
Compensatory hunger refers to higher levels of hunger in response to calorie restriction, which causes people to eat more than they need when at last, they 'allow' themselves to eat.

Research has shown that ADF does not boost compensatory appetite as much as it does the continuous limit on calories. Yes, many people who seek changed ADF say their hunger is through after the first two weeks or so. Some will notice after a while that the days of fasting are almost effortless.

The effects of ADF on hunger, though, are most likely to vary among women.

Alternate-day fasting and body composition

It has been shown that ADF has unique effects on your body composition, both during your diet and during your weight-maintenance period.

Studies comparing conventional calorie-restricted diets and ADF suggest that they are similarly effective at reducing weight and fat mass. Moreover, ADF tends to be more efficient at maintaining muscle mass. This is really significant because losing muscle mass, along with fat, reduces the number of calories.

One study compared ADF to a conventional, calorie-restricted diet that had a deficit of 400 calories. No difference was found in weight recovery between the classes, both after an eight-week analysis and 24 unsupervised weeks. Nevertheless, the ADF group had retained more muscle mass after the 24 unsupervised weeks and lost more fat mass than the calorie-restricted group.

Alternate-day fasting and autophagy

One of the most prevalent effects of fasting on the body is autophagy stimulation.

Autophagy is a process involving the decay and replacement of old cell pieces. It plays a very important role in the prevention of diseases like cancer, neurodegeneration, heart disease, and infections.

Animal studies have consistently shown that long-term as well as short-term fasting improves autophagy and is associated with a delay in aging and reduced tumor risk. Fasting has also been demonstrated to increase lifespan in mice, bees, yeasts, and worms. Moreover, cell experiments have shown that fasting induces autophagy, leading to results that could help keep your body healthy and help you live longer.

Human studies have confirmed this, showing that ADF diets reduce oxidative damage and encourage improvements that may be associated with longevity.
The results look very promising, but ADF's impact on autophagy and longevity need to be investigated in greater depth.

Health benefits other than weight loss

Apart from weight loss, ADF has several health benefits.

Type 2 Diabetes

Type 2 diabetes constitutes 90–95 percent of cases of diabetes in the US. Additionally, pre-diabetes is present in more than a third of Americans, a disorder in which blood sugar levels are comparatively higher than normal but not high enough to be considered diabetes.

Losing weight and reducing calories is typically a successful way of improving or eliminating many Type 2 diabetes symptoms. Compared to continuous calorie restriction, ADF tends to cause slight reductions in risk factors for type 2 diabetes in overweight and obese people. However, ADF seems to be most successful in lowering insulin levels and decreasing insulin resistance. High insulin levels (hyperinsulinemia) have been associated with obesity and chronic diseases. Reducing insulin levels and insulin resistance can lead to a significant reduction in the risk of type 2 diabetes, particularly when combined with weight loss.

Heart health

Heart disease is the world's leading cause of death, responsible for about 1 in 4 deaths. A lot of studies have shown that ADF is a good option for overweight and obese people to lose weight and reduce risk factors for heart disease. Some research on the subject range from 8-12 weeks and are performed in people who are overweight and obese. The most common health benefits are:

1. Reduced circumference of the waist.
2. Blood pressure decreased.
3. Lower concentration of LDL cholesterol (20 to 25 percent).
4. The number of large LDL-particles increased, and the harmful small, compact LDL-particles reduced.
5. Blood triglycerides decreased (up to 30 percent).

Is it good for normal weighted women?

ADF is useful for more than just weight loss— it can also support normal-weight women from health benefits. After a strict ADF diet, a 3-week study examined normal-weight women with zero calories on days of fasting.

Researchers found that it increased fat burning, reduced fasting insulin, and a 4 percent decrease in fat mass. However, throughout the study, hunger levels remained very high, speculating whether a changed ADF diet with one small meal on days of fasting might be more tolerable for normal-weight people.

Another study in both normal-weight and overweight women found that there was a decrease in fat mass following an ADF diet for 12 weeks and positive changes in heart disease risk factors. That said, ADF usually gives you much fewer calories than you need to keep weight, which is why people ultimately lose weight. If you don't want to lose weight or fat mass or continue with underweight, other dietary approaches are likely to match you better.

Eat or not to eat during alternate fasting?

During fasting days, there is no general rule on what you should eat or drink, except that the total calorie consumption should not exceed 500 calories. Drinking low-calorie or calorie-free beverages, such as juice, coffee, and tea, is best on fasting days.
Some people find it best to consume one 'large' meal late in the day, while others prefer eating early or splitting between 2-3 meals. Since your calorie intake will be very limited, focusing on healthy, high-protein foods and low-calorie vegetables is better. Without many calories, those will make you feel whole.

Soups may be a good option on days of fasting because they tend to make you feel more full than if you eat the ingredients alone.

Here are a few examples of meals suitable for days of fasting:
- Eggs and vegetables.
- Yogurt with dried berries.
- Grilled fish with potatoes, or lean meat.
- Soup and a fruit slice.
- A generous lean meat bowl.

Is it safe or not?

Research has shown that, for most women, alternate-day fasting is healthy. It does not result in a greater chance of regaining weight than traditional diets that are limited by calories. On the contrary, long-term weight loss may be even better than continuous calorie restriction. Others claim that ADF increases your risk of binge eating, but studies have found that depression and binge eating have significantly decreased. It also improved the restrictive understanding of eating and body image among people with obesity.

3.5 Warrior intermittent fasting

The Warrior Diet is a way to eat that varies, with short windows of overeating, extended periods of little food intake. It was marketed as an efficient way to lose weight and increase the strength and mental stability levels. Yet some health experts argue that this form of fasting is severe and superfluous.

This segment addresses all you need to learn about the Warrior Diet to help you decide whether it is a safe and effective way to improve your health.

General information about warrior intermittent fasting

This type of intermittent fasting diet is considered a type of intermittent fasting and eating patterns umbrella term that includes periods of reduced calorie intake over a defined period of time. The Warrior Diet is based on ancient warrior eating habits, which ate little during the day and then feasted at night.

It's intended to 'improve the way we eat, smell, act, and look' through stressing the body through decreased food intake, activating 'survival instincts', according to its author. It should be remembered that Ori Hofmekler himself admits that the Warrior Diet is focused on his own convictions and experiences — not solely on research. Under this diet, people undereat for 20 hours a day, then consume as much food as they want at night. Dieters are advised to eat small amounts of dairy products, hard-boiled eggs, and raw fruits and vegetables, as well as plenty of non-calorie beverages during the 20-hour fasting period.

People will literally gorge on any food they want after 20 hours within a four-hour window of overeating. Unprocessed, nutritious, and organic food options are nevertheless promoted.

Does it have benefits?

The Warrior Diet has no research to back up the exact methods, but it does intermittent fasting. Although the Warrior Diet is somewhat more severe than other, more common types of intermittent fasting such as the 16:8 method (fasting for 16 hours and then eating over the remaining 8 hours), this approach is simply a more strict form. Therefore one would argue that the benefits associated with intermittent fasting also extend to the Warrior Diet.

It May Help Weight Loss

Different methods of intermittent fasting have been linked to weight loss, including a 20-hour fasting periods.

One research, which closely mimicked the Warrior Diet (fasting for 20 hours), found that people who ate meals for four hours a night had more weight loss than those who consumed the same amount of calories in meals all day long. What's more, those who eat one meal a day reported significantly reduced fat mass and increased muscle mass. A recent review of six studies found that different types of intermittent fasting, varying from 3 to 12 months, were more successful than no dietary intervention in encouraging weight loss.

Nevertheless, the review found that there were no significant differences in weight loss between dieters using intermittent fasting or continuous calorie restriction (normal diet), which meant that calorie restriction without fasting was equally effective.
However, while the Warrior Diet's most common outcome is to minimize calorie intake, some women adopting this eating pattern may potentially consume too many calories over the four-hour overeating duration, and experience weight gain.

Can Improve Brain Health

The Warrior Diet, as a way to improve brain health, is promoted. Intermittent fasting has been found to support inflammatory pathways controlling that affect brain function.

Animal studies, for example, have shown that intermittent fasting has decreased inflammatory markers such as interleukin 6(IL-6) and tumor necrosis factor-alpha (TNF-α), which may adversely affect memory and learning. Several animal studies found a protective effect of intermittent fasting against Alzheimer's disease. Nonetheless, work is ongoing in this field, and more human studies are needed to establish the effects of intermittent fasting on brain health.

May Decrease Inflammation

Oxidative stress inflammation is believed to be the cause of many diseases, such as heart disease, diabetes, and certain cancers. Studies have shown that intermittent fasting can be an effective way to reduce the body's inflammation. One analysis in 34 healthy women showed that the intermittent form of fasting of 16:8 reduced levels of beta TNF-α and interleukin 1 (IL-1β), substances promoting inflammation.

Another research in 50 women found that those fasting for Ramadan's Muslim women's holiday had significantly lower levels of the IL-6, C-reactive protein (CRP) and homocysteine inflammatory markers compared to non-fasting women.

Fasting Could Improve Blood Sugar Control

Several studies have found that intermittent fasting in those with type 2 diabetes may improve blood sugar control. Research in 10 women with type 2 diabetes found that an 18–20-hour daily fasting target led to a significant decrease in body weight and a significant improvement in fasting and post-meal blood sugar control. Another study showed that intermittent fasting increases the chances of hypoglycemia (low blood sugar), even when taking lower doses of blood-sugar-reducing medicines.

Although it is important to reduce blood sugar levels in a safe manner, hypoglycemia can be harmful and cause serious complications. It is for this reason that women with diabetes who are interested in trying intermittent fasting should first consult their doctor.

Potential downfalls of the Warrior intermittent fasting

Despite the Warrior Diet's potential health benefits, this way of eating does have some declines.

It may be difficult for many women to stick

One of Warrior Diet's most obvious limitations is that it limits the amount of time you can consume regular meals to four hours. It can be really hard to stick to, especially when taking part in normal social events such as having breakfast or lunch.
While some people may feel fantastic when consuming relatively small quantities of calories over a span of 20 hours, others may find that eating this way is not suitable for their lifestyle.

It's unacceptable for a lot of women

This method of intermittent fasting is unacceptable for many women, including:
1. Women who are pregnant or nursing
2. Women with diseases such as type 1 diabetes, heart failure, or certain cancers.
3. Extreme athletic women
4. Women with eating disorders or a history of disordered eating
5. Women who are underweight.

Many women may be able to fast without negative effects intermittently. Some may, however, suffer unpleasant side effects such as insomnia, anxiety, missing periods, and reproductive health disorders.

It Can Lead to Disordered Eating

The Warrior Diet avoids overheating, which can be troublesome for many. Although Ori Hofmekler believes that eating 'when you feel happily happy' should be avoided, this may not translate into healthy eating habits for all. The Warrior Diet may lead to behaviors of binging and purging, particularly those at risk of developing disordered eating. Binging on large amounts of food can also lead to feelings of regret and shame, which can have a negative impact on mental and body image.

Could lead to negative side effects

The Warrior Diet could lead to side effects, some of which might be severe. Potential side effects include:
Fatigue
Dizziness
Low energy
Light-headedness
Depression
Insomnia
Extreme appetite
Low blood sugar (hypoglycemia)
Constipation
Fainting
Irritability
Hormonal imbalance
Weight gain

In fact, many health care professionals claim that dieters will not get enough nutrients if they adopt an intermittent fasting program such as the Warrior Diet. Nevertheless, as long as balanced, nutrient-dense foods are selected, and calorie needs are met, you will meet nutrient needs by carefully preparing your food choices following the Warrior Diet.

How to follow intermittent warrior fasting

Women starting the Warrior Diet will pursue an initial three-week, three-phase plan to improve the capacity of the body to use fat for energy.

Phase I (week one): 'Detox.'

1. Under-eat green juices, pure broth, dairy (yogurt, cottage cheese), hard-boiled eggs, and raw fruit and vegetables for 20 hours during the day.
2. Eat a salad followed by one large or several meals of plant proteins (beans), wheat-free whole grains, small quantities of cheese and cooked vegetables, during the four-hour overeating period.
3. You will drink coffee, tea, water, and small amounts of milk throughout the day.

Phase II (week two): 'Low fat.'

1. Under-eat on vegetable juices, pure broth, milk (yogurt, cottage cheese), hard-boiled eggs, and fresh fruit and vegetables for 20 hours during the day.
2. Eat a salad followed by lean animal protein, cooked vegetables, and at least a handful of nuts, during the four-hour overeating period in the evening.
3. During phase II, no grains or starches are eaten.

Phase III (week 3): 'Concluding Fat Loss.'

This phase varies between high carb intervals and high protein intakes.

High-carb days: 20 hours in the daytime on vegetable juices, clear broth, milk (yogurt, cottage cheese), hard-boiled eggs, fresh fruit, and vegetables. Eat a salad accompanied by cooked vegetables, small quantities of animal protein, and one key carbohydrates such as potatoes, pasta, barley, or oats during the four-hour overeating era.

On high-protein, low-carb days: on vegetable juices, light broth, milk (yogurt, cottage cheese), hard-boiled eggs, and raw fruit and vegetables for 20 hours during the day.
Whole grains or starches are not to be eaten during the overeating window of phase III, a small amount of fresh tropical fruit may be eaten for dessert.
Once the women have completed the three stages, they will start from the start.

What to eat and to avoid?

While dietitians are allowed to eat any food they want, fresh, healthy, organic foods are encouraged, while processed foods, preservatives, added sugars, and artificial sweeteners should be avoided.

During the undereating period, foods to eat in small portions:

1. Fruits: strawberries, bananas, kiwi, mango, peach, pineapple, etc.

2. Vegetable juices: beet, celery, carrot, etc.
3. Bread: Duck, beef, and so on.
4. Fresh vegetables: beans, tomatoes, peppers, onions, mushrooms, etc.
5. Dairy: milk, yogurt, cheese, etc.
6. Protein: Hard-boiled or poached eggs Drinks: beer, seltzer, coffee, tea, and so on.

During the overeating process, foods to eat:

1. Cooked vegetables: cauliflower, sprouts from Brussels, zucchini, spinach, etc.
2. Proteins: Duck, Steak, Salmon, Eggs, Pork, etc.
3. Starches: rice, beans, corn, sweet potatoes, etc.
4. Grains: Oats, quinoa, pasta, barley, potatoes, etc.
5. Dairy: Dairy, cheese, yogurt, and so on.
6. Fats: Olive oil, nuts, etc.

Foods to avoid:

Candies, Cookies, and cakes Chips Fast food Fried food Processed meats (lunch meats, bacon) Refined carbohydrates Chemical sweeteners Sweetened beverages such as fruit juice and soda.

3.6 Tips for maintaining intermittent fasting

Sticking to an intermittent fasting regimen can be difficult. The following tips will help people stay on track and reap intermittent fasting benefits:

1. Stay hydrated. Drink plenty of water and calorie-free drinks, such as herbal teas, all day long.
2. Evicting obsessions with food. Schedule plenty of activities on fasting days to stop thinking about food, like catching up on paperwork or watching a film.
3. Rest and unwind. Evite strenuous activities on days of fasting, while light exercise like yoga may be beneficial.
4. Make a count of every calorie. If the program chosen requires some calories during times of fasting, choose nutrient-dense foods that are rich in protein, fiber, and healthy fats. Beans, lentils, eggs, fish, nuts, and avocado are just some examples.
5. Eat very voluminous foods. Select nutritious and low-calorie foods like popcorn, raw vegetables, and high-water fruits, such as grapes and melon.
6. Raising your appetite without the calories. Generously season meals with salt, herbs, spices, or vinegar. Such foods are relatively low in calories and full of flavors, which can help to reduce hunger feelings.
7. After the fasting period, choose the nutrient-dense foods. Eating high-fiber foods, vitamins, minerals, and other nutrients helps stabilize blood sugar levels and avoid nutrient deficiencies. A balanced diet will also improve weight loss to overall health.

Now, you have learned about almost all the types of intermittent fasting that you can adopt. You should adopt that type of intermittent fasting that your body can adjust to, and that is best for yourself.

In the next chapter, you will read about the myths that you have already heard about intermittent fasting. And you will also learn in the next chapters that those myths are not actually that truthful.

Chapter 4: Things that women need to learn about intermittent fasting

The benefits of intermittent fasting that a body receives from it are numerous. The most noticeable advantage of intermittent fasting is weight loss. Beyond this, however, there are many potential benefits, some of which have been recognized since ancient times. But there are some problems or misconceptions you have to face, too. I addressed all the common myths and difficulties a woman has to face in the intermittent fasting. And there are also many other things you need to know; for example, what a woman should eat or drink during this intermittent period of fasting, or what common mistakes women make during this intermittent fasting which leads to intermittent fasting failures.

4.1 Myths, women hear about intermittent fasting

Intermittent fasting has become common amongst many. Many men and women of all age groups have jumped into this health and fitness trend bandwagon to help them lose weight and improve their health. You want to be sure that you are specific about what this sort of 'diet' actually consists of before you go through the steps of supposed fans. Intermittent fasting has become ever more prevalent. In reality, intermittent fasting is often marketed as a miracle diet, a dietary pattern that varies between fasting and eating times.

Yet not everything you've read about meal duration, and that's true to your wellbeing.

And there are many myths that women have to hear about intermittent fasting. And thus, those myths will be busted at some point.
Following are those myths that you hear all the time:

1. Skipping breakfast makes you fat

One enduring misconception is that breakfast is the day's most important meal. People commonly assume that skipping breakfast leads to excessive weight gain, appetite, and cravings. One 16-week study of 283 people with excess weight and obesity found no difference in weight between those who ate breakfast and those who did not.
Therefore, breakfast does not affect your weight in large measures, although there may be some variation in the person. Several reports also show that people who lose weight, in the long run, tend to eat breakfast. What's more, children and adolescents who eat breakfast tend to perform better in school.

It is important to pay attention to your particular needs as such. For some people, breakfast is helpful, while others can miss it without any negative consequences. Some people can benefit from breakfast, but it is not necessary for your health. Controlled studies indicate little difference in weight loss between those eating breakfasts and those missing them.

2. Consuming also enhances metabolism

Most people think consuming more meals improves the metabolism rate, allowing the body to burn more calories overall. Perhaps your body is wasting some calories digesting meals. This is called food's thermal effect. TEF uses about 10 percent of your total calorie intake on average. What counts, though, is the overall amount of calories you consume— not how many meals you eat.

The result of consuming six 500 calorie meals is the same as eating three 1,000 calorie meals. With an average 10 percent TEF, in both cases, you can burn 300 calories. Numerous studies show that increasing or decreasing meal rates have no effect on overall burned calories. Contrary to popular belief, eating smaller meals doesn't increase your metabolism more often.

3. Feeding also helps to reduce hunger

Some people believe that regular feeding helps to prevent chronic hunger and cravings. Yet the proof is mixed. While some studies suggest that consuming more regular meals results in reduced hunger, other studies have found little effect or even increased rates of hunger. One research that compared consuming three or six high protein meals per day found that eating three meals more effectively reduced hunger.

That being said, reactions will depend on the person. When eating regularly decreases the cravings, this is probably a good idea. Also, there's no evidence that eating or snacking more often decreases everyone's appetite. There is no clear evidence that eating decreases total hunger or calorie consumption more often than not. Alternatively, some studies indicate that smaller, more regular meals increase hunger.

4. Frequent meals will help you lose weight

Since eating more often does not improve your metabolism, it has no effect on weight loss, either. In reality, a study of obesity in 16 adults compared the effects of eating 3 and 6 meals a day and found no difference in weight, fat loss, or appetite. Some people claim eating also makes it more difficult for them to adhere to a healthy diet. Though, if you think eating more often makes eating fewer calories and less junk food easier for you, feel free to stick with it. There's no proof that changing your meal frequency will help you lose weight.

5. Your brain needs a daily dietary glucose supply

Many people claim your brain will stop functioning if you don't eat carbs every few hours. This is based on the belief that only glucose can be used in your brain for food. Your body can, however, easily produce the glucose it requires through a process called gluconeogenesis.

Your body can produce ketone bodies from dietary fats, even during long-term fasting, starvation, or very-low-carb diets. Ketone bodies can feed parts of your brain, significantly reducing its need for glucose. Many people, however, report feeling tired or weak when they don't eat for a while. If that refers to you, think about keeping snacks on hand or feeding more often. Your body will generate glucose to fuel your brain on its own, meaning you don't need a daily intake of glucose in the diet.

6. Eating is often good for your health

Most people think incessant eating is better for your health. Short-term fasting, however, causes a cycle of cellular repair called autophagy, in which the cells use energy from old and damaged proteins. Autophagy can help protect against age, cancer, and diseases such as Alzheimer's disease. Occasional fasting thus has many benefits for your metabolic health.

Many reports also indicate that eating or snacking very often affects your health and increases the risk of getting sick. One research, for example, showed that a high-calorie diet with regular meals resulted in a significant increase in liver fat, suggesting a higher risk of fatty liver disease. Additionally, some observational studies suggest that there is a much higher risk of colorectal cancer in people who eat more often. Snacking is a misconception that it's actually good for your health. Alternatively, from time to time, fasting has significant health benefits.

7. Fasting puts your body in starvation mode

One common argument against intermittent fasting is that it puts your body in hunger mode, thus shutting down your metabolism and stopping you from burning fat. While it's true that long-term weight loss will reduce the number of calories you burn over time, that happens regardless of the method of weight loss you use.

There is no evidence that intermittent fasting brings about a greater reduction in burned calories than other methods for weight loss. In fact, the metabolic rate may be boosted by short-term fasts. This is because of a drastic increase in norepinephrine blood levels, which increases your metabolism and instructs your fat cells to break down body fat. Studies show that fasting can improve metabolism by 3.6–14 percent for up to 48 hours. When you run any longer, though, the results will reverse, weakening your metabolism.

One study showed that fasting for 22 days every other day did not lead to a reduction in the metabolic rate, but on average, a 4 percent loss of fat mass. Short-term fasting doesn't put your body into starvation mode. Alternatively, you increase your metabolism by up to 48 hours during fasts.

8. The body can only use a certain amount of protein per meal

Most people claim you can only digest 30 grams of protein per meal and eat every 2-3 hours to maximize muscle gain. Evidence does not support this, however. Studies show that consuming the protein more often does not affect muscle mass. For most people, the most important factor is the total amount of protein eaten — not the number of meals it spreads over. The more than 30 grams of protein per meal can be easily used by your body. Obtaining protein every 2−3 hours is excessive.

9. Intermittent fasting causes you to lose muscle

Some people believe your body starts burning muscle for fuel while you run. While this generally happens with dieting, no evidence suggests that it occurs more with intermittent fasting than other forms.

On the other hand, studies show that intermittent fasting is effective at maintaining muscle mass. In one analysis, intermittent fasting caused a similar amount of weight loss as constant calorie restriction— but with much less muscle mass reduction. Another study showed a modest increase in muscle mass for people who ate all their calories during one massive evening meal.

There is no evidence to suggest that fasting produces more muscle loss than traditional limits on calories. Studies actually show that intermittent fasting will help you retain muscle mass while dieting.

10. Intermittent fasting is bad for your health

Although reports that intermittent fasting is damaging your wellbeing may have been reported, studies show that it has some significant health benefits. For example, it affects the longevity and immunity-related gene expression, and it has been shown to extend animal lifespan.

It also has major benefits for metabolic health, such as increased insulin sensitivity and decreased oxidative stress, inflammation, and risk of heart disease. It can also promote brain health by increasing levels of neurotrophic factors derived from the brain (BDNF), a hormone that can protect against depression and other mental disorders. Despite the proliferation of myths that it's unhealthy, short-term fasting has important benefits for your body and mind.

11. Intermittent fasting makes you overeat

Some people claim that intermittent fasting causes you to overeat during times of feeding. While it is true that you can compensate for calories lost during a fast by eating a little bit more naturally afterward, this compensation is not total.

One study showed that the next day, people who fasted for 24 hours ended up eating just around 500 extra calories — far less than 2,400 calories they had lost during the fast because it reduces the total rate of food intake and insulin thus improving metabolism.

12. On days off-days, you can eat whatever you want.

Fact: When you surpass your maintenance calories on days off-days, you will not lose weight on fasting diets. You can follow a healthy eating schedule on off days, but you don't have to limit yourself to a set number of calories. I recommend that my patients listen to their hunger instead of weighing and controlling them.

Eat a balanced diet that contains fruits, vegetables, and whole grains to prevent overeating too much. Try lean meats, poultry, fish, beans, eggs, and nuts, if you don't have dietary restrictions. Nevertheless, concentrate on real food. Avoid processed goods, and don't be fooled by marketing claims of 'clean' or 'organic.' Check the list of ingredients for the refined carbs, secret trans fat, chemicals, and added sugars on each bottle.

13. If you start an intermittent fasting program, you're trapped to do it for life

The benefit of intermittent fasting is that it reduces your hunger and cravings. So after you've been without that long enough midnight snack of potato chips or licorice, you won't eventually want it anymore— without having to work hard not wanting it. The trick is to train your taste buds to love good food and avoid foods that are most likely to lead to weight gain and chronic illness.

There are several forms of fasting, and there is evidence that general health and weight management support their effectiveness. Sadly these advantages are often overshadowed by misconceptions promoted by hypotheses that put many off even trying IF.
Intermittent fasting is just one of our recommended dietary strategies. If one is concerned that their current dietary approach

does not allow them to achieve their health goals, they should not be put off trying IF by any of the myths discussed in this book issue.

4.2 Difficulties you have to face during intermittent fasting

As we have discussed how helpful and advantageous is intermittent to our body. So, it also has many side effects as well you and your body need to face. But on this topic, you will learn about the most common things that you definitely have to face during intermittent fasting.

That is:

1. Hunger
2. Dehydration

Hunger and intermittent fasting

You've done your research, heard the stories, and watched people with intermittent fasting change their wellbeing. You are absolutely convinced. Intermittent fasting is a simple solution for safety, wellness, and longevity changes. Yet hold on, one small issue — hunger — is there.

'How can I welcome hunger into my life with pleasure?' Yeah, hunger is part of intermittent fasting, but most probably not the way you see it. If you've ever felt hunger pangs, or 'hanger' (feeling hungry and angry), you may think that this feeling gets ten times worse when you run. This isn't the case. Hunger is fleeting, and will last only about 20 minutes — most people don't know about it, as they don't let hunger last long enough, if at all.

In some situations, people never get to a real hunger state because their appetite keeps them still full. Appetite is an urge to eat that can be caused by hormones, senses (sights, odors, and sounds), or feelings such as hunger and stress. In comparison, real hunger is a physical need to feed, often combined with grumbling stomach and discomfort. This is an important distinction to make, as if you understand why you feel hungry, you will take control of the situation, and your hunger.

The most important thing to understand is that feeling hungry is good, and not being afraid of it. It may feel momentarily awkward, but there will be nothing wrong with it. Hunger is, as Pavlov demonstrated, a conditioned response to a stimulus, which can be reconditioned. For starters, have you ever seen simultaneous hunger strikes, every day?
This is because the hormone ghrelin, which increases appetite, rises in anticipation of a daily meal — at regular feeding times, the body has learned to induce hunger. Clever, huh?!

The initial stages of fasting are probably the most difficult because your' learned appetite' will make you eat, and real hunger will make some use of it. There are many strategies. However, that will help you ride the wave of hunger, comfortably. In this article, I'm going to talk about seven strategies that help manage hunger, so you can achieve your target of intermittent fasting.

1. Cooking low-carb, high-fat

What you eat is just as important as cooking. Know intermittent fasting is not a visa for eating food of poor quality. Alternatively, use that to make the most of your diet and health. High-quality, low-carbohydrate, high-fat, and moderate protein meals between fasts are recommended. This will balance blood sugars, cultivate satiety, and make fasting run smoother.

In general, intermittent fasting is a natural development from a well-established low-carb diet, since reduced appetite is very normal. For whatever cause you're fasting intermittently, a high-fat, low-carb diet can improve your results, help you achieve your health goals faster.

2. Start with low-carb and fat adaptation

Continuing on from above, planning the foundation with a low-carb diet is a good way to start intermittent fasting. Once you're fat-adapted (i.e., use fat effectively for fuel rather than glucose), the appetite will have decreased significantly, and fasting will feel instinctive and effortless. Take at least two weeks to change your diet and consider adding intermittent fasting.

3. Reduce stress, get a good night's sleep and stop alcohol

Poor sleep, stress, and alcohol have a profound effect on appetite as they interfere with the control of hormone and blood sugar. Through improving the quality of sleep, employing stress reduction strategies, and reducing alcohol consumption, these sugar and hormone-induced hunger pangs can be sided.

Make sure your bedroom is comfortable and well ventilated to improve sleep quality; adhere to a normal bedtime, which is not too late; block noise and light; do not eat at least 3 hours before bed; avoid screens and blue light an hour before bedtime; wind down with a book; add exercise to your day.

Sure, a good night's sleep will have a positive effect; knocking on your stress levels. You can also practice stress management strategies such as yoga, meditation, exercise, journaling, and counseling for an extra bit of relaxation and serotonin (the happy hormone).

In order to prevent unstable hormones and blood sugars, try to limit alcohol consumption as much as possible, but particularly the day before a fast. If you want to drink alcohol, you should reasonably choose the low-carb choices in moderation. Our alcohol guide should clarify in greater detail.

4. Keep hydrated

Thirst can often be mistaken with a sense of hunger, so hydrate yourself with plenty of water. Get a head start on hydration and try drinking 1 to 2 glasses of water when you wake up first. Look for about 2–3 liters, total every day— drinking too much water will flush out valuable electrolytes, so don't overboard.

Drinking water can also offer physical fullness filling that will help with real hunger pangs. Whatever hunger you feel, water is your tool at fasting. If you find it difficult to drink water, especially in the morning, try adjusting the temperature, making it more appealing, depending on your preference for warm or chilled water. Instead, if that doesn't work, you can try sparkling water with an infusion of mint and lemon.

5. Replace the electrolytes and consume salt

The loss of electrolytes during intermittent fasting is a typical and natural reaction. As a result, given your attempt to drink gallons of water, you can feel dry mouth and thirst. Such symptoms can make you feel thirsty and hungry (as described earlier, thirst can often be confused with hunger).

Electrolytes are important to health and wellbeing, so we advise you to stay in top condition until symptoms occur. You should liberally drink bone broth and salt food during your eating time to replace the electrolytes. Additionally, a supplement of magnesium and potassium may be helpful (you should take these while fasting). Here's our electrolyte guide, which will go through it in greater detail.

However, a pinch of salt is a perfect way to clean the palate and dampen hunger. Use a little bit at a time, a few dabs on your tongue, and let it work its magic — hunger will disappear in no time, along with that awful coating in your mouth.

6. Drink a coffee or tea

Fill the void with a freshly brewed, black tea, or coffee. Unlike drinking water, a hot drink will give you a sense of fullness, but will also take on the role of 'hand-to-mouth,' making you feel like you've eaten.

Try bulletproof drinking coffee — coffee with added fats such as butter, coconut oil, MCT oil, and ghee if you're really dealing with hunger and intermittent fasting. By preserving ketosis and autophagy, the fat will keep you full— two primary mechanisms that underpin fasting and its benefits. For the purist fasting, eating a single calorie can break a fast, but if adding fat to your coffee means you stick with a fast, or find it easier, then I'd say it's worth it 100 percent.

7. Distract yourself

Organize exercise, sports, and seeing friends while you normally eat or when there is hunger. Like we spoke about earlier, the ghrelin levels will rise at mealtimes, so get ready and make sure you have something fun to do around these times. You're going to be so nervous about enjoying yourself that ghrelin-induced hunger can come and go without even noticing you. Nonetheless, whatever you do, don't let yourself get bored, as we all know, this is an easy pass to get hungry into!

Plan for famine, but don't be afraid. I tell you, the hunger isn't going to be as bad as you think. With these tips and tricks under your belt, you can easily cast aside hunger pangs and achieve your target of fasting.

Bear in mind that our programmed appetite is impaired by fasting, so the easier it becomes, the more you do it. Fasting will be an instinctive, natural part of your day before you know it, as you respond to the rhythm of true hunger, rather than appetite. When hunger feels too daunting, you may need to change your fasting regime with all that said. Fasting should be relatively easy, relaxed, and suitable for your life.

Dehydration and intermittent fasting

During intermittent fasting, it is surprisingly easy to become dehydrated. You might probably need to drink water more often than you would think. Remember this: you hydrate the most when feeding, like fruits and vegetables, either from a bottle or from the water-dense foods on your plate. So, dehydration during intermittent fasting is definitely a risk, considering that between these occasions, you have fewer meal opportunities and potentially day-long stretches between.

You can and should still be drinking water during those fasting periods. Water needs differ depending on the individual, but 2.2 liters for women and 3 liters for men are a good rule of thumb. Our real need for hydration is higher, but about 20 percent of it is met by food, provided we eat enough fruits and vegetables. This window is a modal one.
Staying hydrated is always vital; however, when your food intake is usually reduced, it is even more so during intermittent fasting. Around 20 percent of our daily intake of water comes from food. So, drinking more when you're fasting is especially important. One of the side effects you may suffer from intermittent fasting is a headache. Although it may occur for several reasons, dehydration is one of the most common.

To get all of the Intermittent Fasting's health benefits, such as fat loss, increased metabolic rate, lower blood sugar rates, improving the immune system, and so on, you need to limit the intake of any fatty food. But you can still eat non-caloric beverages because they don't break your fast and encourage you to get all the fasting benefits. This is because non-caloric drinks do not induce insulin release, and as a result, do not interfere with fat burning and autophagy.

In fact, the benefit of consuming plenty of liquids while fasting intermittently–it can help you overcome hunger during your fasting period. But the question is, what are you allowed to drink during intermittent fasting so as not to break your fast? So exactly what to drink while fasting?

Mineral water

Can you drink water while fasting?
No... YES. Mineral water and vapor are usually calorie-free and are permitted during fasting. Mineral water is mineral-filled to help restore the electrolyte and mineral imbalance that occurs when fasting. For this reason, the most recommended Intermittent Fasting drink is mineral water.

Coffee

Coffee is permitted during the hours of fasting, and, in addition, several studies have shown that it can help fat burning and reduce the sensitivity to insulin over time. It also serves as an appetite suppressant for many people and is, therefore, a good choice for those hungry fasted mornings.
Nonetheless, too much caffeine can have a harmful effect on your body, so don't overdo the recommended daily dosage of 400 mg (2-2.5 cups of brewed coffee) for healthy adults.

Apple cider vinegar

Apple cider vinegar (ACV) is calorie-free and allowed during fasting. Generally, it helps to lower blood sugar levels and improve digestion after Intermittent Fasting.
How to put it to use? Drink 1-2 tbsp of distilled apple cider vinegar in beer. Specifically, drinking it before a meal will improve digestion and increase the sense of fullness.

Stevia

Stevia is a natural sweetener, and a good choice if you need a sweet thing. Research has shown that compared to artificial sweeteners, it has no negative side effects and may even prefer levels of glucose and insulin. Nonetheless, it could instigate some hunger, and you might want to be careful.

Coconut oil

Pure fats include coconut oil, MCT oil, and other oils. Technically speaking, anything that has calories breaks your strong even if it's a tiny amount. Nevertheless, fat has little to no effect on insulin, blood glucose, or any of the other tests that suggest a 'broken fast.' As popularized by Bulletproof fasting, coconut oil could, therefore, be considered a part of fasting.

Nonetheless, if you prefer' natural' fasting (something we suggest for our 21 Day Intermittent Fasting Challenge), you can try to keep up with any oils and/or butter consumed. Meaning-no Bulletproof coffee during the hours of your fasting. Please remember that fats are incredibly high in calories, so if you're trying to lose weight, you should keep this in mind.

Butter

Butter is pure fat, similar to coconut oil. It also has little to no effect on insulin and may be tolerated when fasting (e.g., drinking bulletproof coffee). Unlike coconut oil, however, it is extremely high in calories, and therefore not recommended for our 21 Day Intermittent Fasting Challenge.

Almond milk

Breaks the almond milk a fast? Technically, Yes, Hell! But if you really have to have something and are OK with' free fasting' coffee with almond milk, splash can be a good alternative.
Almond milk is low in carbs and calories, so a good vegan choice for' safe intermittent fasting' could be up to 0.5 cup/100 ml of almond milk. If buying almond milk, avoid those with added sugar, or those with extra protein fortified.

Bone broth

Bone broth is usually very low in calories and carbs but contains a protein that breaks down quickly, fat burning, and autophagy technically. Nevertheless, some experts allow bone broth on exceptional cases (up to 20 kcal per fasting period), especially since it helps to replenish the lost salt while not eating.

Artificial sweeteners

There is a lot of conflicting information and various studies conducted around artificial sweeteners and their health and insulin response effects. While some studies show that artificial sweeteners like aspartame, saccharin, or sucralose do not elevate insulin, in some people, they may disturb the balance of gut bacteria.

Given the uncertainty and ongoing discussions about the impact of artificial sweeteners, we recommend that you avoid artificial sweeteners at all. The most popular artificial sweetener brand names include Splenda (sucralose), Nutrasweet, Equal or Sugar Twin (aspartame), Sweet'N Low (saccharin).

From the previous topic, you have learned about what to drink during intermittent fasting. Now, you are curious to know what you should eat during intermittent fasting. If you want to know about this, then you have to read the next topic.

4.3 What should women eat during intermittent fasting?

While the word 'fasting' sounds frightening, intermittent fasting (IF) takes the diet world by storm. With a fair amount of research on the positive impact of the diet on body weight, memory, and blood sugar, it's no wonder that the IF bandwagon seems to be running to everyone you meet. Perhaps the appeal is the lack of rules governing food. When you can eat, there are limits but not exactly what you can consume. So should you be downing ice cream pints and chip bags while fasting intermittently? Likely not. Eating at intermittent fasting is more about being balanced than just dropping your weight quickly. Therefore, selecting nutrient-dense foods such as vegetables, fruits, lean proteins, and healthy fats is critically important.

The list of intermittent foods to fast should include:

1. For protein

Protein Recommended Dietary Allowance (RDA) is 0.8 grams per kilogram of body weight. Depending on your fitness goals and level of activity, your requirements can differ.

By reducing energy intake, increasing satiety, and improving metabolism, protein helps you lose weight. In fact, heightened protein intake helps build muscle when combined with strength training. Getting more muscle in your body naturally increases your metabolism because your muscle absorbs more calories than fat. Included in the IF protein food list is: poultry and fish Eggs Seafood Dairy products such as milk, yogurt, and cheese Seeds and Beans and legumes Soy Whole grains.

2. For carbs

According to American Dietary Guidelines, 45 to 65 percent of your daily calories should come from carbohydrates. Carbs are your body's principal source of energy. The other two comprise protein and fat. Carbs come in different shapes. The sugar, protein, and starch are the most important.

Carbs often get a bad rap because they cause weight gain. All carbohydrates, however, are not created equal and are not necessarily fattening. Whether you're gaining weight or not depends on the type and quantity of the carbohydrates you eat.
Make sure you pick foods high in fiber and starch but low in sugar. A study carried out in 2015 indicates that consuming 30 grams of fiber every day can cause weight loss, raise glucose levels, and lower blood pressure. Having 30 grams of your dietary fiber isn't an uphill struggle. They can be obtained by consuming a basic egg sandwich, Mediterranean chickpea rice, peanut butter apple, and enchiladas with chicken and black peas. The IF Carb Food List includes Beetroots sweet potatoes Quinoa Oats Brown rice Bananas Mangoes Apples Berries Kidney Beans Pears Avocado Carrots Broccoli Brussels sprouts Almonds Chia Chickpeas seeds.

3. For fats

For Americans, fats will contribute 20 percent to 35 percent of your daily calories according to the 2015-2020 Dietary Guidelines. Saturated fat should not contribute more than 10 percent of daily calories, most notably.Depending on the type, the fats can be healthy, poor, or simply in between. Trans fats, for example, increase inflammation, reduce the 'healthy' cholesterol levels, and increase the 'bad' cholesterol levels. They're used in baked goods and fried foods.

Saturated fats can increase cardiovascular risk. Expert opinions on this vary, though. Eating these in moderation is appropriate. Red meat, whole milk, coconut oil, and baked goods contain high saturated fat content. It contains monounsaturated and polyunsaturated fats. Such fats will lower the risk of heart disease, lower blood pressure, and lower blood fat levels. Rich sources of these fats are olive oil, peanut oil, canola oil, safflower oil, sunflower oil, and soybean oils.

4. For a healthy gut

A growing body of evidence indicates that the secret to your overall health is your gut health. Billions of bacteria known as the microbiota are in your gut. Such bacteria affect the health of your body, your metabolism, and your mental health. These may also be involved in many psychiatric conditions. So, you should look after those tiny bugs in your stomach, particularly when you are fasting intermittently. The intermittent fasting food list for a healthy gut includes All vegetables, Kefir Kimchi, and Fermented Vegetables.

In addition to keeping the gut safe, these foods can also help you lose weight by:

1. Reducing fat absorption from the stomach.
2. Increase excretion of ingested fat through stools.
3. Reduce dietary intake.

5. For hydration

According to the National Academies of Sciences, Engineering and Medicine, the average requirement for women, about 11.5 cups (2.7 liters).

Fluids include water and water-containing foods and drinks. During intermittent fasting keeping hydrated is important to your health. Dehydration can give rise to headaches, extreme fatigue, and dizziness.

If you are already dealing with these fasting side effects, dehydration can make them worse or even more severe.

Foods to exclude from the intermittent fasting food

- Processed foods
- Refined grains
- Trans-fat
- Sugar-sweetened beverages
- Candy bars
- Processed meat
- Alcoholic beverages

4.4 Mistakes that women usually make during intermittent fasting

Many people come into trouble with Intermittent Fasting when they approach it in the wrong way, being conscious of the right approaches can be the difference between success and failure when performing Intermittent Fasting. Here are the top five errors women make when they're fasting all the time:

1. An excuse to eat rubbish

Sadly, people think that intermittent fasting is a magic pill that fixes all their problems. Sure, taking control of your health is an incredibly effective method, but eating a diet full of processed foods and sugar won't be canceled. It's even more important to feed your body with nutrient-dense, whole foods when you are intermittent fasting. The body begins to break down damaged components when you are in the fasted state and then uses them for energy, this cycle cleans and restores the body. It also means that your body becomes more receptive to the food you eat, this is fantastic if the body is full of nutrients, but not good if you eat garbage! Not only that, if you don't feed on nutrient-dense foods, you're going to feel hungry all the time–your body's going to be missing nutrients.

2. Try to restrict calories during the 'food window.'

One of the main problems some people face when they start IF is that they want to restrict calories when they break their quick. In this way, the whole idea to eat is to listen to your body and start eating until you feel full. Your body is an incredible machine if you let it do its job properly. Your body will release hormones that will make you feel complete when you know that you've had enough food. When you limit calories during your eating time, you can end up eating, which causes a lot of unhealthy changes in your body and is not good for you in the long term.

3. Make sure you eat the correct amount of calories for fat loss

Try to do too many things at once–by train, exercise, and try fasting. If you've spent a few years eating poorly and not exercising and you'd like to try IF, don't bite off more than you can chew (pun intended!) at the beginning. Facilitate yourself slowly in fasting and exercise; do not start training five days a week, fast regularly, and limit calories from day one when you eat. The combination can give rise to adrenal fatigue. Your body thrives here and there with a little physical stress, but too much stress can turn into a problem. The simplest and most effective tool for intermittent fasting weight loss success

4. Obsessing about timings and 'food windows.'

In my view, one of IF's main advantages is to allow you to be completely in sync with your body and appreciate what I call' true hunger'–something that occurs every 16-24 hours, not every 4 hours. When you should eat your body should decide, not the clock. When you concentrate on periods of time, you end up counting down the hours until you can feed-you never learn to understand messages from your bodies. You choose to miss either breakfast or dinner with The 2 Meal Day; by doing so, you stretch your overnight fast to about 16 hours. The emphasis isn't on the time period; you can break your fast anytime you feel hungry if you choose to miss the meal.

93

5. Not drinking enough water

Once the body is in a fasted state, the weakened components start to break down and detoxify the body. It is very important that you use drinking lots of water to flush out those toxins. Ideally, you'll be drinking more water than you would usually. I drink about 4-5 liters a day, most of that during my time of fasting. Not only that, drinking water, particularly sparkling water, will help you feel complete, which is crucial when you get into intermittent fasting first.

In the next chapter, you will learn about how to get started with intermittent fasting.

Chapter 5: Transitiong into intermittent fasting

Intermittent fasting is a powerful tool for blood sugar control, insulin sensitivity enhancement, and diabetes reversal. It's been getting a lot of support lately, quite simply because it works and it's fast.

You have read earlier about the choices you can take for intermittent fasting, so as you know that there are many different ways of fasting so that everyone can have things in their lives in some shape or form. Now the question arises what those things you need to consider before taking any kind of intermittent fasting.

There are a number of reasons people run, ranging from religious traditions to medical procedures to wanting to drop those last two pounds before slipping into a wedding dress. Yet, without instructions, fasting should not be taken lightly or gone through. Every day, your body is used to eating nutrients from food and drinks, and cutting them off fully comes as a shock to your system.

Many people are just shocked by how much fasting interferes with their ability to perform their daily tasks. Others are shocked that fasting doesn't help them achieve their desired results. If you are fasting it for religious reasons, you will be more pleased with the experience, and at least less humiliated if you are doing it for physical reasons, if you are able. Here are the first things you need to know before fasting.

Ease Into It

Unless you've ever fasted before, do not start with a seven day fast. Start with a conventional fast within 24 hours, then move it up to three days if the first one goes well. With the time-limited method, don't restrict yourself automatically to eating eight hours a day, if you're used to eating every hour you're awake; continue for 12 hours on, 12 hours off, and go from there. Have realistic expectations, and progressively change your current routine.

Plan Ahead and Be Flexible

Once you're accustomed to fasting, you may find that you can install a short quick on a little notice. But when you're starting out, make sure you plan your fast at least a couple of days ahead. You'll want to make sure your quick doesn't interfere with work, family, or training, all of which can negate the test run's positive effects.

Have some thought into where you are going to be fasting and how. Quick home before you try it out in the woods or on holiday. Got plenty of water at hand. Tell your friends and family that you're fasting, and they know what's going on if you start feeling irritable, so at the next group dinner, you won't have to answer the same questions twenty-five times.

Don't be too stiff

When you normally eat from 11 am. Eating before a morning sprint or a major day of training, closing the fasting window, is perfectly fine before 7 a.m. Consistency is good; that is not inflexibility.

Prepare for Your Body to Feel Different Most people feel drained, get a headache, and usually feel 'out of sorts' on any fast days two or three. It is natural. Usually, by the end of day three or four, the negative side effects of fasting are gone away. If you go less than two days, you'll probably start feeling better just as the fast comes to an end. When you turn the corner on day three after the negative symptoms have passed, most people feel great, and a sense of calm, well-being, and increased concentration takes over. But if during a fast — more than just feeling a little tired — you feel like something is wrong definitely eat. You can always try another time again.

Talk to your doctor before starting

In particular, if you have any medical conditions or are on any medication.

Last but not least, just keep it simple

 Fasting (in this experiment) is defined as consuming only flat or carbonated water, or black coffee, or unsweetened tea. Continue to consume your normal meals when watching the food. Intermittent fasting works best in my personal experience when paired with a low-carb-high-fat diet of whole organic foods. But it's not your goal right now to launch the perfect combination to get the best results... it's a fast finish.

In the following chapter, you will study about the steps you have to take in order to do intermittent fasting:

5.1 Learn about your natural eating pattern

Awareness is the very first step towards any change in diet. You should start paying attention to what you eat and start to be aware of your dietary choices. This will serve you well during your intermittent rapid feed periods. It's a well-known fact that one of the easiest ways to change unhealthy eating habits is to track the foods you consume first, when and how much.

Writing them down in a small notebook is the best way to keep track of these. Carry a pen and paper, or make notes about when and what you eat in an app on your phone or laptop. Many people are shocked by the amount of food they eat in a day. The recognition of specific eating patterns and preferred food types is the right place to start when embarking on intermittent fasting.

Create a food journal or log (you'll find a link in the bonus section to get a copy of a free printable food journal) that includes the following items:

1. **Log the Date and Day of the Week:** Remember whether it's morning, noon or night. Once you start fasting, you will need to be time-specific.

2. **What are all the foods and beverages consumed:** list the kinds, quantities, and whether you used condiments, butter, sugar, etc. to add calories. Beverages count, so make them think too. Keep notes of what you add as a sweetener to your drinks, such as sugar or honey. This will later become significant.

3. **Portion sizes:** The length, weight, or a number of items figures work just fine. Whether you like weighing, that's perfect too. It is about getting a sense of quantity.

4. **Your meal location:** take notes of where you're at mealtime. Are you at a desk or on a sofa? Should you feed by yourself or with others?

5. **What is the extent of your eating activity:** pay attention to what you concentrate on as you eat food. Are you surfing the web or checking out Facebook, or just talking to friends?

6. **How do you feel:** What are your feelings? Are you full of happiness, enthusiasm, depression, tension, anxiety, or content? Our emotions can drive our food choices, and eating can trigger emotions in the opposite direction. Pay particular attention to eating changes based on emotional situations.

To make your dietary journal useful, be open and honest. Take the time to take note of every bite of food you eat and drink. You won't have an accurate picture of your dietary habits if you don't log everything in. Seek to monitor your food intake within 15 minutes of the time you eat for the correct results.

Use a 7-day daily food log. They should not be days in a row. The aim is only to get an illustration of what your natural food tendencies and preferences are. This will provide the knowledge you need later on about your habits and will serve the purpose of acclimating your mind to the role of being mindful of what you are eating, where, why, and how you feel.

It is not necessary that you consume a perfectly balanced diet, but good choices will be of good service. There are whole books written about what's best to eat. Try eating a well-balanced diet with plenty of whole grains, beans, fruits, and protein. Try to limit sugar and processed foods. Include healthy fats for beneficial nutrients, like those present in olive oil, almonds, avocados, and whole milk products

The next step is how to choose an intermittent fasting plan that suits your lifestyle.

5.2 Choosing a fasting plan

Intermittent fasting is a powerful tool for blood sugar control, insulin sensitivity enhancement, and diabetes reversal. It's been getting a lot of support lately, quite simply because it works and it's fast.

There are different ways of intermittent fasting so that everyone can take some form or form in their lives. With that said, finding the right regime for fasting that fits into your life is important. No way to quick is wrong or right, but the right way for you to melt into your routine, encourage a productive day, and feel sustainable.

This topic will address several aspects that are worth considering when selecting a lifestyle-fitting fasting schedule. You can then start tailoring a fasting program to suit your needs and life with all things considered.

What is the schedule for your work, and when are you busiest?

Plan your fasts for your schedule — easy when you're short on time and save food when you've got more time to prepare and digest. The morning is an optimal time to fast for most people since this is usually the busiest time of day.

Not only will you gain some extra time by skipping a meal or two, but productivity will also improve. Fasting greatly improves concentration and concentration, and your to-do list will fuel you with turbo. Additionally, the fasting process will be made easier by a busy work schedule. Your mind is going to focus on things other than food that will help make hunger blunt.

When will you eat with your family and friends?

Sitting down and eating a meal with family and friends is vital for your wellbeing. Choose your fasting time when you are less likely to eat with others — maybe this is the a.m. when everyone runs out of the house, or maybe at night when people are busy with activities.

Whether you normally eat breakfast, lunch, or dinner with your friends and family, keep this as part of your day and easy around the day. It's precious to eat & spend time with people.

When are you usually hungry, or are you eating the most?

Do you eat a king-like breakfast, a prince-like lunch, and a pauper? Or does that early food thinking make you feel queasy? Follow your appetite and what feels right for you.

Despite popular belief, there is no need for breakfast. You're not in the mood for food when you wake up, then eating your first meal later in the day is perfectly acceptable (and encouraged). Similarly, if your appetite naturally tapers towards the end of the day, then seek to miss your meal in the evening.

Focus your eating window around your hungry appetite— this will be different for everyone.

Are you going to exercise?

Fasting and exercise are complementary to each other, so set a fasting schedule during exercise. Fasting increases exercise performance and outcomes because exercise enhances the benefits of fasting (autophagy, glucose removal, etc.) — diet can also be used to boost your fasting regime— it keeps your mind off food and serves as a suppressant of appetite.

When you usually practice breakfast in the morning, postpone it until later. When you work out at night, start and stop eating earlier in the day so you can work out with an emptier stomach.

What are your priorities and objectives, and where are you on your health care journey?

Determine where and what you want to do in your wellness journey. If you're new to intermittent fasting, or you're not yet adapted to fat, then slowly ease into it. You can do this by growing your normal eating window every day by half an hour before you hit a time frame with which you are relaxed.

Alternatively, if you were looking to reduce blood sugar or reset your appetite quickly, it might work well for a 24–72 hour fast. A long fast is an excellent way to reduce glucose and move the body quickly to ketosis, however demanding they are.

If you're a seasoned intermittent faster, looking to kick off a fat loss plateau or move your fasting schedule to the next level, then pursuing longer fasts on a weekly, monthly or annual basis might be a good option.

Remember, there's nothing in stone Life is chaos, and it's new every day

Similarly, the fasting scheme should be versatile enough to switch through your schedule every day. Nothing is set in stone, and breaking your fast an hour earlier than intended is absolutely fine — it will not impact your score.

Giving yourself the freedom to fast by lifestyle and how you feel is likely to lead to better adherence. Just being more aware of the signs of hunger and knowing when you start and stop eating is a gentle and efficient way to introduce fasting into your daily life. Instead of following intermittent fasting as a rule book, make it a natural extension that enhances your daily lives. There's something for everyone, so discover what fits well for you, and have fun experimenting.

After choosing your plan for intermittent fasting, you have to follow this thoroughly. When you are following your plan of intermittent fasting, you have to consider the following things:

1. Listen to your body
2. Eat healthy in between
3. Last but not least, you should know when to quit.

Chapter 6: Side-effects that women face by Intermittent fasting

Intermittent fasting is one of the most trendy diet plans of the moment, both evangelized by actors from Hollywood, execs from Silicon Valley, and influencers from Instagram. Its followers forego food from 16 hours to a whole day anywhere, with many swearing by its weight loss, brain enhancement, and other benefits.

Yes, recent studies suggest intermittent fasting can help you shed pounds and stave off a host of chronic illnesses, including heart disease, diabetes, Alzheimer's disease, and cancer. Some even point to its life-extending ability. But the experts we consulted note that these results come with caveats: most work on intermittent fasting has been conducted on animals, and the few human studies out there have mainly looked at health indicators (such as glucose levels) rather than actual health effects (such as diabetes) and only lasted a few months.

In many cases, the negative side effects of fasting may outweigh any potential benefit. Here are some signs an irregular pattern of fasting is dangerous or harmful.

6.1 You might experience hormonal imbalances

Several women who were attempting to undergo intermittent fasting skipped periods, metabolic disturbances, and even early menopause. Sure, for some women, this can work. But here is why intermittent fasting can be detrimental, even harmful, to your goals. Intermittent fasting is the custom of long periods without food.

There is evidence that if IF done appropriately, blood glucose can be regulated, lipids can be managed, corona disease risk reduced, the weight of the body can be maintained, lean weight gained (or retained), risk of cancer reduced, and much more. It was in the mid-20s in women as young.

Intermittent fasting and female hormones

Experimenting with IF seems tiny in the grand scheme of health decisions you make in your life, right? Sadly— at least for some women— it seems small decisions can have big impacts. The hormones that control key functions such as ovulation are incredibly sensitive to your energy intake; it turns out.

Hypothalamic-pituitary-gonadal (HPG) axis — the joint activity of three endocrine glands — acts a bit like an air traffic controller, in both men and women. Next, the hypothalamus activates hormone-emitting gonadotropin (GnRH).

It signals the transfer of luteinizing hormone (LH) and follicular stimulating hormone (FSH) to the pituitary. Both LH and FSH function upon gonads (a.k.a. testes or ovaries).

In women, this stimulates estrogen and progesterone development — which we need to release a mature egg (ovulation) and support a pregnancy. This in men stimulates testosterone production and sperm output. Because this chain of reactions happen in women on a very complex, regular cycle, GnRH pulses have to be timed very precisely, or anything can get out of whack. GnRH pulses tend to be highly sensitive to environmental factors and can be thrown away by fasting.

In some women, even short-term fasting (say, three days) changes hormonal pulses. There's even some evidence that skipping a single regular meal (while not constituting an emergency by itself, of course) will start putting us on alert, perking up our antennae so that our bodies will be ready to respond rapidly to the change in energy intake if it persists. Perhaps this is why some women are doing IF just fine while others are running into problems.

Why does intermittent fasting affect women's hormones more than men's?

We are not absolutely sure. Kisspeptin induces the development of GnRH in both sexes, and we know it is very responsive to leptin, insulin, and ghrelin— hormones that control and respond to hunger and satiety.

What is noteworthy is that female mammals have more kisspeptin than males. More kisspeptin neurons can mean greater sensitivity to the energy balance changes. This may be one reason why fasting makes women's production of kisspeptin dip more readily, tossing their GnRH off-kilter.

Fertility, metabolism and intermittent fasting

You might think: Well, what's the big deal if kisspeptin falls off and I miss a couple of periods? I'm not getting children anytime soon, anyway. Here's the stuff. The metabolism and the female reproductive system are deeply intertwined. If you're skipping cycles, you can bet a lot of hormones have been interrupted— not just those that help you get pregnant. Women used to eat less protein than men in general. Obviously, female fasts should eat even less. Less protein consumption means taking in fewer amino acids.

The activation of estrogen receptors and the synthesis of the insulin-like growth factor (IGF-1) in the liver involve amino acids. IGF-1 causes thickening of uterine wall lining and menstrual cycle development. Low protein diets can, therefore, reduce fertility. However, significantly, it is not just for reproduction that estrogen is.

All over our bodies, we have estrogen receptors, including in our hearts, GI tract, and bones. Change the hormone level, and you change the physiological process all over: memory, moods, metabolism, regeneration, protein turnover, bone formation... estrogen functions in a few ways when it comes to appetite and energy balance.
First, estrogens change the peptides in the brainstem, which signal that you feel full (cholecystokinin) or hungry (ghrelin). Estrogens also stimulate neurons in the hypothalamus.

Do something that causes your estrogen to drop, and you may find yourself feeling a lot more hungry — and eating a lot more— than you would normally. And estrogens are essential regulators of metabolism. Yes, pluralist estrogens. Because, over time, the estrogenic metabolite ratios (estriol, estradiol, and estrone) change. Estradiol is the big player, until menopause. It decreases after menopause, while estrone remains about the same.

It remains unclear the precise functions of each of these estrogens. A drop in Estradiol may cause fat storage increases. Why? For what? Since Estradiol is made using fat. This can explain in part why it's harder for some women to lose fat after menopause. And it

could serve as a reason to take care of your reproductive health —
even if you're not focused on making babies.

How does your body know?

Women's hormonal equilibrium is especially sensitive to how
much, how often, and what we eat. But how does that 'know' our
bodies when food is scarce?
It was the proportion of a woman's body fat that controlled her
reproductive system. The theory was that if your fat reserves
dipped below a certain percentage (a reasonable guess might be
around 11 percent somewhere), hormones would get messed up,
and your cycle would end. Boom: No risk of becoming pregnant.

That makes quite a lot of sense. When there is not much to eat, you
will, over time, lose body fat. But in fact, the situation is more
complicated than that. Food availability can change rapidly, after
all. And — as you probably know, if you've ever attempted weight
loss — it often takes a while to lose body fat, even if you're eating
fewer calories.
In the meantime, women who are not very lean may also stop
ovulating and lose their cycles. That is why scientists have come to
believe that for this cycle, the overall energy balance may be more
important than the amount of body fat percentage.

Stressors and energy balances

In fact, the negative energy balance in women may be due to the
hormonal domino effect of which we have been talking.
The effect can be negative energy balance: too little food, poor
nutrition workouts too much stress disorder, illness, chronic

inflammation too little rest and rehabilitation Hell; we can even use energy reserves when trying to keep warm.

Any combination of these stressors could help to place you in a negative energy cycle and avoid ovulation: marathon training and flu nursing; too many days in a row at the gym and not enough fruit and vegetables; intermittent fasting and busting your butt to pay the mortgage.

You wonder, did she just pay the mortgage by reference? You're Betting. Psychological stress can play an essential part in destroying our hormonal balance.

Our bodies can't tell the difference between our thoughts and feelings, creating a real threat and abstract stuff. The stress hormone suppresses the production of estrogen and progesterone in the ovaries. Meanwhile, during stress, progesterone is converted to cortisol, which means less progesterone, which contributes to the domination of estrogen in the HPG axis. You could be 30 percent fat floating. But if your energy balance has long enough been negative, particularly if you are depressed, then reproduction stops.

Anyway, that's the idea.

What to do now?

Intermittent fasting is likely to affect reproductive health based on what we know if the body sees it as a major stressor. Whatever affects your reproductive health can affect your overall health and fitness even if you don't even plan on having babies. Yet periodic procedures for fasting differ with some being far more severe than others. And things like your age, nutritional health, the length of time you're fasting, and other pressures in your life— including exercise— are also likely important.

So, so. Were you fasting?
Bearing in mind how much remains unclear, If you want to try IF, begin with a gentle procedure and watch out for the way things go.

Do not start intermittent fasting:
1. When your menstrual cycle ends or becomes erratic
2. When you have trouble falling asleep
3. When your hair falls out when you begin to develop dry skin or acne
4. When you find that you don't recover from workouts as quickly
5. When your injuries are slow to heal, or
6. When any bug goes around, your resistance to stress decreases your mood when your heart starts swinging.

6.2 General side effect that you will face

You've learned so much about the benefits of intermittent fasting (IF), including weight loss, decreased inflammation, enhanced digestion, decreased bloating, increased mental control, improved sleep, and a handle on sugar cravings. You've learned so much about the benefits of intermittent fasting (IF), including weight loss, decreased inflammation, enhanced digestion, decreased bloating, increased mental control, improved sleep, and a handle on sugar cravings.

You're ready to try it out, but you need to be mindful of some not-so-awesome side effects of the gene that you'll probably encounter in the beginning.

Hunger

When you're used to eating five or six times a day, at certain times, your body comes to expect food. The hormone ghrelin is charged with making us feel hungry. It usually occurs at breakfast, lunch, and dinner, and is partly controlled by the intake of food. The ghrelin levels will tend to rise when you start fasting first, and you'll feel hungry. It will take serious will-power at first. When you hit the beginning of your eating period, and you don't even feel hungry, a time will come.

Dr. Luiza Petre, a dietary and weight loss expert and board-certified cardiologist, recommends battling hunger in the first or two weeks by consuming tons of water to keep your belly full, making you feel more alert and satiating the habit of having to put something in your mouth. Pound at least 1 liter within 30 minutes of waking up. Drink another liter or more if you experience a pang of hunger. One thing you'll know from intermittent fasting is that what you felt was hunger was actually thirst or boredom.

Cravings

If I told you couldn't eat watermelon again, odds are, you'd just want to eat a slice of watermelon. You are going extra long stretches without eating during intermittent fasting. And chances are, you can just think about eating. That is when the anxiety sets in. You will also find that you are more likely to crave sweets and refined carbohydrates because your body is searching for that hit of glucose. Do whatever you can not think about food, and be sure to indulge yourself a little while during your feeding time so that you can fulfill those cravings.

Headaches

Dull headaches that come and go are quite normal as the body gets used to this new eating routine. Dehydration can be one reason, so make sure you drink tons of water during your fasting and feeding windows.

Low Energy

Your body doesn't get the constant source of fuel you used to consume all day long, so expect to feel a bit sluggish during the first few weeks. Try to keep your day as comfortable as possible, so that you can expend as little energy as possible. You may want to give a break to your workouts or just do light workouts like walking or yoga. Gaining extra sleep will help, too.

Feeling irritable

Feeling hungry is true and sucks. Watch for a little cranky when the blood sugar levels drop, or you're struggling with IF's other side effects, such as cravings and low energy.

Heartburn, Bloating, and Constipation

Your stomach generates acid to help digest your food, so you may feel heartburn when you're not eating (this side effect isn't as common as the others). This could range from mild discomfort to full-on pain, to burping all day. Time is supposed to cure this side effect, so just keep drinking water, prop up while you sleep, and avoid greasy, spicy foods when you eat that could make your heartburn even worse. If this isn't going away, talk to your doctor.

Intermittent fasting can also lead to constipation, which can lead to bloat and pain. Stephanie offers to make you drink tons of water.

Feeling Cold

Fasting cold fingers and toes are pretty common, but for a good reason! If you fast, the flow of blood to your fat stores' increases. Called blood flow of adipose tissue, this helps move fat into your muscles, where it can be used as a fuel. That can also make you more susceptible to feeling cold when your blood sugar falls. Beat the cold by sipping hot tea, taking warm showers, wearing extra layers, and avoiding long periods of time outside in the cold.

In the next chapter, you will read about when a woman should avoid intermittent fasting.

Chapter 7: When women should avoid intermittent fasting?

For some people, a complete game-changer is intermittent fasting (IF). It's the secret to everything from successful weight loss to increased mental focus to a significant energy boost.

Nevertheless, just because for some people, intermittent fasting is the go-to lifestyle doesn't mean it's for every woman. While intermittent fasting is quite a healthy choice for some, it can, in fact, be dangerous for others. But, who should exactly avoid intermittent fasting? What are some of those hazards?

Insulin-Dependent Diabetic Women

Women who are dealing with type 1 or insulin-dependent diabetes are those who may place themselves at serious risk by pursuing an intermittent fasting regimen. Intermittent quick intervals between fasting times and uncontrolled feeding. This could be very dangerous in women with diabetes and who take anti-diabetic medications, particularly insulin. In the days of fasting, anti-diabetic medicines, specifically insulin, will continue to have an effect on blood sugar. That could drop the levels of sugar to a dangerous point. Diabetics need steady levels of blood sugar to stay healthy (via both diet and exercise). For intermittent fasting, that can be almost impossible.

Endurance Athletic women

Are you training for a marathon? If so, it probably isn't intermittent fasting for you. Nutrient timing is extremely important for sports success and, when adopting an intermittent fasting diet, would be a challenge. Because of the excess calories consumed, endurance sports need increased calorie needs. And, the effect[that] endurance exercise on nutritional requirements requires regular calorie intake and sufficient macronutrient intake before, during, and after an event or long training session to rebuild muscle, replenish glycogen reserves, and maintain electrolyte balance. Intermittent fasting doesn't offer you a steady dose of nutrients and calories you need to prepare, perform, and heal. So, if you have an endurance event coming up, you will prepare to stop intermittent fasting.

Women with a history of disordered eating

If you are healing from disordered eating habits, intermittent fasting is a no-go. Women who want to stop intermittent fasting include those with a propensity to an eating disorder or an eating disorder history. Intermittent fasting includes periods of restriction followed by periods of consuming larger meals. In people who struggle with limiting, binging, or other disordered eating patterns, this can be particularly disturbing. It is safer in such situations to stop intermittent fasting entirely and to adhere to a more stable nutrition plan.

Pregnant women

If you are carrying a child, you must adopt a nutrient-filled pregnancy diet (and calories!) to keep your baby and you healthy.

Unfortunately, with intermittent fasting, you won't get that — women who are pregnant and breastfeeding due to increased calorie and nutrient needs. If you are pregnant, you need to eat often enough to help your baby and your safety. The intermittent fasting system just doesn't allow for that.

In the next chapter, you will read about the most common pros and cons of intermittent fasting.

Chapter 8: Pros and cons of intermittent fasting

There are many pros and cons regarding intermittent fasting that a woman should know. It will guide you properly about the intermittent fasting.

Following are the most common pros of intermittent fasting, that you may have already read about but here is a light sneak peek on it:

Easy to follow

Many dietary patterns focus on eating specific foods and limiting other foods or avoiding them. Learning a particular eating style rules may require a substantial commitment of time. There are entire books dedicated to explaining some form of intermittent fasting.

On a meal plan that includes intermittent fasting, you simply eat depending on the time of day or day of the week. Once you've decided which intermittent fasting regimen is best for you, all you need to know when to eat is a watch or a calendar.

No Calorie Counting

Not surprisingly, women who try to achieve or maintain a healthy weight generally prefer not to count calories. Although nutrition labels can be found easily on many foods, the method of calculating portion sizes and tabulating daily counts can be tedious either manually or with a smartphone app.

Intermittent fasting is a simple alternative where it needs little or no calorie-counting. Calorie restriction (and subsequent weight loss) occurs in most circumstances because food is either eliminated or significantly restricted on certain days or during certain hours of the day.

No Macronutrient Limitations

Common eating plans are in place, which significantly restricts different macronutrients. Many women, for example, adopt a low-carb diet plan to boost health or lose weight. Many follow a low-fat diet for medical purposes or for weight-loss.

Each of these programs allows the user to adopt a new way of eating — often substituting favorite foods for fresh and probably unknown foods. This may require new cooking skills and learning to shop differently and store the kitchen.
During intermittent fasting, none of these skills are needed, simply because there is no goal macronutrient spectrum, and no macronutrient is limited or prohibited.

Unrestricted eating

Any woman who has ever changed her diet to achieve a medical benefit or a healthy weight knows that you are starting to crave foods that you are advised not to consume. Nevertheless, a study published in 2017 indicated that an intensified desire to eat during a weight-loss journey is a key factor.

Yet, on an intermittent fasting schedule, this challenge is strictly limited. Food restriction only happens during certain limited hours, and usually, you can eat whatever you want on the plan's non-fasting hours or days. In reality, sometimes, the researchers call these days 'feasting' days.

Continuing to eat unhealthy foods may not, for example, be the healthiest way to gain benefits from intermittent fasting, but cutting them off during those days restricts the total consumption and eventually may bring benefits.

Could theoretically improve longevity

As discussed before, longevity is one of the most frequently cited advantages of intermittent fasting. Rodent studies have shown, according to the National Institute on Aging, that when mice have put on programs that severely restrict calories (often during periods of fasting), many have shown an extension of lifespan and reduced rates of several diseases, particularly cancers. So, is that profit extended to women? It does, according to the ones promoting the diets.

Following are the cons of intermittent fasting:

Reduced physical activity

One significant side effect of intermittent fasting can be physical activity reduction. A provision for physical activity is not included in most intermittent fasting programs. Not surprisingly, those who follow the programs may feel ample exhaustion to fail to meet their daily goals, and may even adjust their regular exercise routines.

Severe Hunger

Not surprisingly, it is normal for those experiencing severe hunger in the fasting stage of an IF eating plan. This hunger may become more intense when there are others who consume traditional meals and snacks around them.

Medications

Many women who take medicines find it helps to relieve certain side effects by taking their prescriptions with food. In addition, some medications bear the warning that they should be taken with food. Hence it may be a challenge to take medicine during fasting. Before beginning an IF regimen, any woman who takes medication should speak to their healthcare provider to make sure the fasting stage does not interfere with the efficacy or side effects of the drug.

No Emphasis on Nutritious Eating

Most intermittent fasting programs' pillar is pacing rather than food choice. Therefore no foods (including those lacking good nutrition) are avoided, and no foods are promoted, which provide good nutrition. That is why diet-followers do not always tend to eat a healthy diet.

When you follow a short-term, intermittent weight loss fasting regimen or receive a medical benefit, you are unlikely to learn basic healthy eating and cooking skills, including how to cook with healthy oils, how to eat more vegetables, and how to pick whole grains over refined grains.

May Promote Overeating

Most intermittent fasting protocols, meal size, and meal frequency are not limited during the' feasting' period. Consumers then enjoy a diet on ad libitum. Sadly, some women can find this encouraging overeating. For example, if after a day of complete fasting, you feel deprived, you may feel inclined to overeat (or eat the wrong foods) on days where 'feasting' is permitted.

In the next chapter you will read about the do's and don'ts that women should follow for intermittent fasting.

Chapter 9: The do's and don'ts of intermittent fasting

In recent years, there have been many exciting developments around the principle of intermittent fasting (IF). Many people are swearing about decreasing body fat, increasing energy and focus, detoxifying, aging, and even protecting them by intermittent rapidly against chronic disease. Nonetheless, intermittent fasting can be shown to reduce the risk of certain conditions, such as type 2 diabetes, heart disease, and even cancer.

Yet, when the discussion comes up about fasting, there's a big question that emerges, particularly as it concerns women: Is it safe for women and their hormones? Let's look at it closer.

Do keep a track on your hormone health

With intermittent fasting, the biggest risk women face is their hormones. Our hormones perform a very delicate balancing act over a regular (on average) 28-day period. Sometimes the slightest change in our diet, wellbeing, attitude, environment, exposure to contaminants, or stress level can cause hormonal imbalance, leading to further health problems along the way. If not done properly, intermittent fasting may easily become one of those hormonal imbalances causes because of the stress on your body that it can create.

Taking the steps listed below will help to keep your hormones controlled, and your stress level regulated tremendously. It's also very important to check your hormone state before you even start.

If you are already struggling with any form of hormonal imbalance, the intermittent fasting program will need to be followed by addressing that issue. Check both your normal cortisol levels and a salivary sample of your monthly hormonal cycle.

Don't diet while fasting

Are you ready for the biggest reason why DOESN'T work for women on intermittent fasting? Because at the same time we try to diet too! This is not the idea behind intermittent fasting and eventually can result in either bingeing, disappointment, or nutritional and hormonal problems. You need to eat over a period of time you are consuming. In that timeframe, eat a lot of really nutrient-dense, caloric-dense foods and don't want to be in a massive calorie deficit. That is not going to work. I like to see intermittent fasting as a healthier, easier, smarter way to reduce calories. Yet, definitely never do the two.

Do keep the focus on fats.

The diet will consist primarily of healthy, nutrient-dense fats to ensure that you do not experience a too high-calorie deficit. Fat from well-reared animals, gross cocoa and coconut oil, nuts and nut butter, butter and ghee, milk, avocado and avocado oil, olive and olive oil, as well as herbal dairy products. You can be sure that in your day before your fast, you get enough nutrients and calories when these foods are a staple.

Not only that, but moving to a high-fat diet will also ensure your times of fasting are stress-free, safe, and comfortable. The blood sugar will become extremely stable, with the reduction of carbohydrates and the addition of a significant amount of fat.

Rather than being a rollercoaster (which is what happens to our blood sugar when our diet includes extra carbohydrates), it will be more like small waves. If our bodies are on the rollercoaster path, a few hours after your last meal, there will be a drop in blood sugar, which will trigger feelings of hunger. Cortisol–the stress hormone–will come to the rescue if no glucose is given through a meal. So, now you're hungry, for another 5 hours you're still fasting, and your body feels a stressful event. Not good.

The body has learned to run on fats-both food and body fat processed-rather than just waiting for the next meal. Not only are you not feeling hungry now, but you're avoiding the stressful event! And, as we discussed above, it is because of the hormonal imbalance that can arise from stress and cortisol response that the reason intermittent fasting can be difficult for women. We just removed the stressor by eating high-fat and plenty of food!

Don't work intensively

For the first of two weeks, at least until you know how erratic that will affect you. When your body is accustomed to this adjustment, chances are workouts in the fasted state will actually feel better, and you will begin to see changes in your workouts. But first, as your body adapts and gets used to this new energy source (fat), you need to remove all the added stressors. Taking nature walks or a really nice yoga class will be the best way to get exercise in during this time of transition. After that, start implementing fast HIIT exercises in the gym such as jumping rope, sprinting, or heavy lifts and see how you feel. Remember, the end goal is to keep your body's stress level at an all-time low, thus keeping your hormones in balance. Exercising too intensely when the body transfers energy sources would likely cause tension.

Do a slow start

In reality, women may be luckier in easing their way into it. Spend 3-4 weeks at first getting fat-adapted with a high-fat diet. To add, as it comes naturally to you, in an intermittent fasting schedule. If you like it to add as you feel comfortable in more days.

Do enlist professional support.

You should also need to seek the help of a specialist to direct you through the improvements you wish to make and to support you along the way. This will make it easier to recognize what's right for you, rather than merely guess.

The last and the next chapter is all about the women above 40 years old or above 50 years old. Is intermittent fasting good for them or bad for them?

Chapter 10: All about middle-aged women and intermittent fasting

This chapter will hold the information about all the effects of intermittent fasting on middle-aged women that are explained below in two sections:

a. Women above 40 years old

b. Women above 50 years old

10.1 Women above 40 years old

You have heard of intermittent fasting, but maybe you are not aware of the many different types. Or the best forms of intermittent fasting for women over the age of 40. Intermittent fasting's most common excuse is to lose weight, and it works, but it also has a lot of other health benefits.

These days, all the cool kids are doing it, but what is it and what are the right kinds of intermittent fasting for women over 40? Fasting may sound difficult, and if you say 'I can't do that' to yourself, I'm here to reassure you that you can, and you are already.
You don't eat when you're asleep, right?

The best intermittent fasting forms for women above 40 are as follows:

16/8 Method

It is one of the most popular methods for intermittent fasting. The 16 reflects the 16 hours you run, and the 8 is the period of time you eat. Only imagine, if you sleep a full 8 hours, you get half of your 16 hours of fasting. Then you can decide if you want to keep fasting once you wake up or stop eating 8 hours before you go to bed (or whatever your number is).

Create a plan and then stick to it. One of my favorite pieces of this kind of intermittent fasting is that you can drink calorie-free drinks like coffee (yay coffee!), wine, and tea.

Do not hesitate if you are a coffee drinker or a tea drinker. When you're getting used to drinking them black, it's not that bad. Nonetheless, watch your intake of caffeine, because it can disturb your appetite or give you the jitters.
Talk to your doctor first before you try this intermittent fasting process.

Alternate Day Fasting (ADF)

You go without eating solid foods for a whole day. But, on fasting days, some people add up to 500 calories. You can drink non-calorie drinks all the time, just like the 16/8 process.

One study revealed that in balanced and overweight adults, ADF is effective for weight loss and heart health. But sustainability isn't easy, and women with specific health conditions may not benefit from this. If you're new to intermittent fasting, this isn't the best strategy either. Instead, you can ease your way into this and continue using the 16/8 process.

Alternate day fasting encourages weight loss but is related to appetite, which can combat weight loss as successful.
Speak to your doctor before you try this more intense intermittent fasting process.

The 5:2 fasting

The 5:2 diet is another type of intermittent fasting, often referred to as The Fast Diet. Ironically this does not involve full fasting. The 5 reflects the five days of the week you're following a normal diet. And the 2 is the two days of the week when you limit your calories by 25%. If your normal calorie consumption is 2,000 calories a week, then on your two days of fasting, you will consume 500 calories per day.

There are no restrictions on what you can eat, so you can easily follow this diet. Health News Today advises that the 2 'fasting' days be spread apart, so they are not consecutive. Which gives your body the calories and nutrients it wants every other day, at least. This diet is simple and versatile to follow. For most, this is very helpful and will not make you feel like you're missing out. This is because you know you will be able to return to your regular eating schedule tomorrow. Talk to your doctor before you try this more intense intermittent fasting process.

Form of fasting will you choose?

These are just three of the many forms of sporadic fasts out there. The 16/8 process, Alternate Day Fasting, and the 5:2 diet are fast and safe ways for those of us over 40, to lose weight.
I strongly advise starting with the 16/8 method. This is because sticking to it is easy, so you'll have better weight loss luck. You

should try Alternate Day fasting and/or the 5:2 diet once you get used to intermittent fasting and see which one is most effective for your body. Until starting with your doctor, some form of intermittent fasting test.

10.2 Women above 50 years old

Intermittent fasting took the world of diet and nutrition by storm, but if you're a woman over 50 years old, is it right for you?
Higher appetite, achy joints, decreased muscle mass, and even sleep problems are some things that make it harder to lose weight after age 50. At the same time, losing weight, particularly dangerous belly fat, can significantly reduce your risk of severe health problems such as diabetes, heart attacks, and cancer.
The risk of developing certain diseases rises as you age, of course. In some cases, intermittent fasting for women over 50, when it comes to weight loss and reducing the chance of usually developing age-related diseases, may function as a virtual youth fountain.

Does fasting work intermittently?

Intermittent starvation, also referred to as IF, isn't going to force you to starve. It also does not grant you permission to consume tons of unhealthy food during the period you're not fasting. Instead of eating all-day meals and snacks, you're consuming within a specific time span.

Most people make an IF schedule, which requires fasting for 12 to 16 hours a day. They eat normal meals and snacks throughout the rest of the time. It doesn't sound as hard to stick to this eating time because most people sleep about eight of their fasting hours. You're also encouraged to enjoy zero-calorie drinks, such as water, tea, and coffee.

You should develop an eating schedule that will work for the best intermittent fasting outcomes for you. For example:

• Twelve-hour fasts: you might just skip breakfast with a 12-12 fast, and wait until lunch. When you prefer to eat your meal in the morning, you will have an early supper and avoid snacks at night. Older women find it rather easy to stick to a 12-12 fast.

• Seventeen-hour fasts: With a 16-8 IF cycle, you will enjoy quicker results. Many people choose to eat two meals within an eight-hour window, and a snack or two a day. You might set your eating time between noon and eight in the evening, or between eight in the morning and four in the afternoon, for example.

• Five-two schedules: Limited eating times may not work daily for you. Another alternative is to fast for five days, stick to a twelve-or sixteen-hour schedule, and then relax for two days. You could use IF during the week, for example, and normally eat on the weekend.

• Another option requires very few calories on alternating days. For instance, on one day, you could keep your calories below 500 and then eat normally the next day. Remember that frequent IF fasts never claim a low-calorie restriction.

As with any diet, if you're consistent, you'll get the best results. At the same time, on special occasions, you should definitely give yourself a break from this kind of eating routine. To find out which kind of intermittent fasting works best for you, you can experiment. With the 12-12 program, lots of people ease themselves through IF, and then they advance to 16-8. You should then try to stick to that strategy as much as you can.

What makes Fasting Intermittent Work?

Many people think IF succeeded for them simply because of the small eating window, of course, allows them to reduce the number of calories they consume. Instead of consuming three meals and two snacks, for instance, they may find they only have room for two meals and one snack. We become more mindful of the types of food we consume and tend to stay away from processed carbs, unhealthy fats, and empty calories. You can, of course, choose the kinds of healthy food you love too. While some people opt to decrease their total intake of calories, some combine IF with a keto, vegan, or another diet.

Benefits of Intermittent Fasting for Women That Extend Beyond Calorie Restriction

While some nutrition experts claim that IF works only because it allows people to limit food intake naturally, others are not in agreement. We claim intermittent fasting results with the same amount of calories and other nutrients are higher than conventional meal plans. Reports have even shown that abstaining from food is more than just limiting the number of calories you consume for several hours a day.

These are some of the metabolic changes that IF induces which could help to account for synergistic benefits:
• Insulin: lower insulin levels can help improve fat burning during the fasting period.
• HGH: HGH levels rise while insulin levels drop to promote fat burning and muscle growth.

• Noradrenaline: the nervous system sends this chemical to cells in reaction to an empty stomach to let them know they need to release fat for fuel.

Is intermittent fasting safe?

Remember, you're only expected to run for twelve to sixteen hours and not at a time for days. You still have plenty of time to enjoy a balanced and fulfilling diet. Some older women may need to eat frequently due to metabolic disorders or medication instructions, of course. In that situation, you can speak to your health care provider about your eating habits before making any changes.

Although it is not strictly fasting, during the fasting period, some doctors reported intermittent fasting benefits by making such easy-to-digest foods as whole fruit. Changes like these can still provide needed rest for your digestive and metabolic system. For example, 'Fit for Life' was a popular book on weight loss, which suggested eating fruit only after supper and before lunch.

In fact, the writers of this book said they had patients with this twelve-to seventeen-hour 'apple' fast each day that just changed their eating habits. We didn't follow the other rules of the diet or count calories, and they still lost weight and become healthier. The approach may have succeeded precisely because the dieters were replacing junk food with whole food. People found this dietary change to be effective and easy to make anyway. Traditionalists won't call this fasting, but it's important to know that if you can't absolutely abstain from food for several hours at a time, you may have options.

Typical Intermittent Fasting Results

Dr. Becky, a chiropractor and fitness consultant over 50, says it is difficult to find any IF downsides in the medical literature. She clarified that your blood sugar and insulin levels would go down to low levels during the fasting period. Without the hormonal fat-storing signal of insulin, the body must rely on energy for stored fat.

You can also find a summary released by the National Library of Medicine of the intermittent findings related to women's health. Several highlights of this study include research on using fasting as a method for reducing the risk of cancer, diabetes, and other metabolic diseases, as well as heart disease.

Is Fasting the Right Fat-Loss Option for You?

In any case, IF seems to work mostly because it is relatively easy for people to stick to. We claim that by eating times, it allows them to reduce calories naturally and make better food choices. Many studies suggest IF is better than just cutting calories, carbohydrates, or fat because it seems to encourage fat loss while maintaining lean muscle mass.

Of course, with another weight-loss program, most people use IF. For example, you might decide to lose weight by eating 1,200 calories a day. In two meals and two snacks, you may find it much easier to spread 1200 calories than three meals and three snacks. If you've been struggling with weight loss because either your diet didn't work or was just too hard to stick to, you could try intermittent fasting for quicker results.

Dr. Kathryn Waldrep suggests eating within a nine-hour window and selecting the time frame depending on the circadian rhythms of your body in Prime Women's recently launched PLATE weight management program. Early risers can eat from 9:00 am until 6:00 pm. At noon, night owls will eat their first meal and finish their last meal at 9:00 am. As more and more research has been done on IF and circadian rhythms, there seems to be credible evidence on the soundness of this weight management approach to eating.

Become a member of PLATE today and take advantage of our special offer if you want to join other women over 50 in a healthy weight loss program combined with intermittent fasting.

Conclusion

Intermittent fasting is a way to move from time to time. It is a common way of losing weight and improving health today.

It might be an ancient secret of wellbeing. It is old because in all human history it has been studied. This is a secret, because until recently this mighty habits, especially regarding our health, had largely been overlooked in many ways. But many are now rediscovering this culinary custom. Since 2010 there have been about 10,000 percent increase in online searches for 'intermittent fasting.' Most have increased in recent years. Intermittent fasting could be of enormous benefit if done correctly, including reduction of excess weight, type 2 diabetes reversal, and many other things. Plus, it can save you money and time.

It appears to be one of the best ways to lose weight, become lean and fit. Intermittent fasting has slowly gained momentum for women as more and more people are becoming aware of its benefits.

This helps to increase energy levels and to improve endurance. Best of all–results hold you inspired. Your cognitive function is said to be enhanced too. But many people continue to be skeptical about the method's effectiveness, as it is not for everyone. Although the majority of women find shorter fasting periods healthy, the extended ones are not recommended for certain women.
The overall advantages of women for intermittent fasting include: improved lean, muscular growth, increased energy, consistent weight loss, increased cell stress reaction, reduced inflammation,

and oxidative stress, enhanced insulin sensitivity in overweight women; and decreased cognitive function due to increased active nerve growth factor.

The first is the fasting stage that causes leptin and ghrelin to produce–starvation hormones.

The second factor in women's sporadic fasting is rapid capacity, so it is not recommended for pregnant women to fast. If a faster woman does not eat enough calories, she may have issues with fertility. Furthermore, there is no need to worry if IF is done correctly. Women may even increase their fertility after losing some overweight.

Intermittent women-fasting can be very helpful if done correctly. When calories are too severely limited, this can cause imbalances in hormones that lead to issues such as infertility and irregular periods. Therefore women who choose to do intermittent fasting should pay attention to their diet's nutritional value. Otherwise, they will lose the IF advantages and offer their bodies more harm than good.

And there are also many options of intermittent fasting that any woman can adopt, but there are some women that need to avoid intermittent fasting at all cost. Those are pregnant women, athletic women, diabetic women, and any women that need more calories per day.

There are also some pros and cons regarding intermittent fasting that women need to learn before starting intermittent fasting. And there are also many side effects that you need to face during intermittent fasting such as hunger, dehydration, constipation, hormonal imbalances, and headache.

References:

Gini Health Blog - Gene Stories. Intermittent Fasting & Its Science Based Benefits. [online] Available at: https://blog.ginihealth.com/intermittent-fasting-and-its-science-based-benefits/.

The Kettle & Fire Blog. 27 Facts about Intermittent Fasting For Women [Healthier & Empowered]. [online] Available at: https://blog.kettleandfire.com/intermittent-fasting-for-women/.

Should Women use Intermittent Fasting For Fat loss?. [online] Available at: https://fityourself.club/should-women-use-intermittent-fasting-for-fat-loss-60b7ef2f69a6.

Intermittent dieter. Debunking 14 myths about fasting and keto - Intermittent dieter. [online] Available at: https://intermittentdieter.com/debunking-14-myths-about-fasting-and-keto/.

2 Meal Day. Is Intermittent Fasting Safe for Women?. [online] Available at: https://2mealday.com/article/intermittent-fasting-safe-women/.

Center For Discovery. The Dangers of Intermittent Fasting - Center For Discovery. [online] Available at: https://centerfordiscovery.com/blog/the-dangers-of-intermittent-fasting/.

Mark's Daily Apple. Should Women Fast?. [online] Available at: https://www.marksdailyapple.com/women-and-intermittent-fasting/.

Healthline. Intermittent Fasting For Women: A Beginner's Guide. [online] Available at: https://www.healthline.com/nutrition/intermittent-fasting-for-women#getting-started.

Medical News Today. Intermittent fasting for weight loss: 5 tips to start. [online] Available at: https://www.medicalnewstoday.com/articles/324882.php#summary.

www.ingramcontent.com/pod-product-compliance
Lightning Source LLC
Chambersburg PA
CBHW031233250726
48655CB00005B/1934